FAT ATTACK

FAT
ATTACK

NARDIA
NORMAN

CONTENTS

RECOVERY

MINDSET

WHAT NOW?

THE FOUR STAGES OF BECOMING A FAT LOSS WEAPON

INTRODUCTION

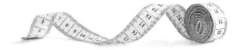

If you've picked up this book, then you're someone who is seeking to make a positive change, to become the person you are destined (and deserve!) to be; one who is a healthier, fitter, stronger, more motivated version of your current self.

So let me start off by saying 'congratulations' on being an action taker! Choosing this book is the first step towards making a significant and permanent change.

Achieving a positive change is not always easy. In fact, when dealing with fat loss, it can be extremely challenging! There is so much confusing information out there about the best way to lose weight, the newest 'pill/potion/magic formula' for dropping the kilos fast, there are 'superfoods' 'good foods' and 'bad foods', and there are a million and one different exercise programs aimed at giving you 'abs in seven minutes' or 'a perky butt in just three minutes a day'. And what is touted as 'good' for you one day, can often be rubbished the next. This overwhelming abundance of information can, understandably, be very confusing.

Then, of course, you add to that confusion the everyday demands such as managing a family, work and having a social life. Trying to do the things you need in order to shed the weight can often feel so daunting, it's no wonder that fat loss gets filed in the 'too hard basket'.

The bottom line is we are fat. And not just a little bit fat, but grossly fat. So much so that obesity has been labeled *the* disease of modern times, responsible for many major health-related problems such as heart disease, kidney failure and diabetes, to name a few.

The strain that an obese and overweight population places on societal infrastructure is enormous, and has many far-reaching implications and complications.

The alarming thing is that obesity is a preventable disease; one that can be manipulated, changed and permanently improved by making changes to one's lifestyle.

Most of us are aware of these worrying statistics so why is it then, that more than half of Australia's population are overweight and more than a quarter are obese? Of course, these figures are not exclusive to Australia; they are reflective of a worldwide trend and are only going to worsen in the future.

There are a host of factors that contribute to this epidemic, including increased access to sugary, fatty processed foods, accessibility to transport, economics, changes in perception of public safety, increased reliance on prescription medication and general lack of desire to take ownership of one's health. The question that needs to be answered is 'how can this be helped?' Or, perhaps a more important question, is 'how can I help you?'

The answer, my friend, lies in the following pages.

For years I have heard people say the same thing over and over again: 'losing fat and creating a healthy lifestyle is too hard'; however it doesn't need to be. In fact, with some simple guidelines, losing fat effectively and, most importantly, for the rest of your life can – and will – be achieved.

Now don't get me wrong, there are still going to be 'tough times', but I am going to share with you the key things needed in order to make permanent fat loss and a healthy lifestyle become your new reality.

The key is to keep taking action. It doesn't matter how small your actions are initially, you just need to keep the momentum going. Small positive changes repeated over time equals big rewarding changes in the long term!

A client of mine, who has since become a very dear friend, came seeking my help after he felt he'd exhausted all other fat loss avenues. The first time I met him he was 27 years old and weighed 268kg. For him, at this point in time, death was a very realistic prognosis and most likely in his very near future.

I know him as Kev, but you may recognise him as 'Big Kev' from the television show *Australia's Biggest Loser*. To date, he has been the show's heaviest contestant – worldwide!

For Kev, everyday tasks were difficult. This included breathing, sleeping, and simply moving from one spot to another. The daily functions that we all take for granted were very hard and time consuming for him to execute. In his words he felt life was 'one big obstacle.'

However, just like anyone, he had to make the conscious decision to take action towards improving his life. He didn't launch himself into a crazy, unrealistic regime; he simply started by making small changes that, over time, resulted in big change. He followed and applied my key rules for long term fat loss and, as a result, is a shadow of his former self. In fact, he is half the man he used to be – literally!

Throughout this book I am going to show you how Big Kev applied my Fat Loss Secrets, in order for him to achieve such a tremendous and impressive transformation – both physically and emotionally.

Kev would cringe hearing me say this, but if Kev can do it, then so can you! Even if your goal loss is 5kg, 10kg, 20kg or 100kg, the time is right for you to make the same life transformation and start living a life you've always dreamed of.

Okay, time for a reality check. I hold both a professional and moral obligation to tell you the truth, so that you are no longer confused or misguided by the ton of B.S that surrounds fat loss and the ways to achieve it. The truth is this. Despite what marketing companies or television shows tell us, there is no one singular, specific methodology that will work for everyone. However, what *does* work is applying a variety of principles and adjusting each one to suit *your* body and individual situation. The fundamental principles that I will provide in this book, is the foundation that you will need to tweak and then apply to suit you.

What this means, is that in order to become a fat burning weapon and transform your life, you must become an expert in YOU!

Becoming an expert in you, involves learning more about yourself and taking responsibility and accountability for your actions. You are in control and, therefore, only *you* can make the necessary changes to achieve your goals.

Your timing is perfect; you are reading this because NOW is right time for you to make the same life transformation that

Kev has achieved. Now is the time for you to finally put yourself first and become the person that you know you are capable of, and deserve to be. This is the first step in your journey.

It is time to become awesome.

HOW TO USE THIS BOOK

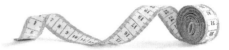

Unlike at school, where you have to read a book from the start to the finish, in this book you may prefer to jump around to any chapter and read it in whatever order you like. Most likely, you'll feel some chapters resonate with you more than others, and some you may find yourself returning to repeatedly. All of this is completely okay. What I do ask of you, however, is that you make the commitment to apply *all* the elements you come across – even the ones that seem difficult.

At the conclusion of the book I have outlined the 4 Stages of Fat Loss, which show you how to implement your new knowledge in a safe and effective manner. Each stage builds upon the previous one, and in order to achieve the long term fat loss you desire, you must take the time to fully embrace and apply the action points at each stage.

One of the biggest secrets for success is understanding that losing fat is a process and not something that should happen overnight. There are many actions that need to be completed in order for you to achieve your goal, and it is the consistent application of the steps I've outlined, that will guarantee your success.

Be aware that your journey is going to be a learning process. There will be lots of habits that you will need to unlearn, and lots of new information and 'truths' to re-learn. Typically, those who are open and willing to learn about themselves, and about nutrition, training, sleep and mindset, are the ones who are most successful at achieving permanent transformations.

My Fat Loss Process has been specifically designed so that all the elements complement each other. In order to maximise your fat burning potential and gain best results, you should focus on improving a habit from each area. The reason for this is because my process takes a holistic approach to fat loss and health. This is why it has worked so well for Kev and my other clients. In fact, while it is possible to lose fat *without* improving your health, at the end of the day any fat loss would be temporary. Long term, sustainable fat loss occurs really only after you have addressed and improved your overall health.

Despite what some may say, good health and fat loss can – and do – belong together.

To achieve long-term fat loss, you must understand there is a strong relationship that exists between nutrition, training, sleep and mindset and, normally, if one is affected, then so too are the others. You have probably experienced this yourself.

If you have had a terrible night's sleep, you are a lot hungrier and crave sugary or salty foods and/or caffeinated drinks to give you the bursts of energy you need to make it through the day. The result of this action is often a 'tired but wired' feeling of jittery anxiousness, which makes it hard to focus on any task, and you feel super tired all day. But, when bed time rolls around again, your mind is still racing and sleep feels like it's miles away.

During days like this it can feel harder to find the motivation and the energy to do something physically active. And because of those cravings, sticking to a healthy eating plan for the day becomes an even more challenging task. What typically happens next is that the interconnected downward spiral continues to the point that all elements become negatively affected: poor nutrition, poor (or no) physical activity, poor sleep and, not surprisingly, a poor mindset.

However, as much as this sounds like doom and gloom, it can be completely reversed. When all these elements are worked on, and good habits are established across all of them, the effects become cumulative. When you eat well, you feel better, when you feel better you do more, and when you do more, you feel good, and so on.

This Fat Loss process is NOT a quick fix – it will take time. But that is not to say you won't experience certain 'quick wins' along the way! Keep in mind that the process is building a new and healthy body that you will live in for the rest of your life – so taking the necessary time and making the sacrifices required will be well worth it in the end.

Along the way, you can find supplementary information such as videos, bonus material and additional support at my website www.nardianorman.com

For best results you can use this book in conjunction with the website, as your 'go-to' for all things related to fat loss and health.

FAT LOSS MYTHS

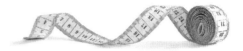

Before we launch into the nitty gritty, I would like to debunk a couple of the biggest myths in the weight loss and fitness industries. It is because of these myths that the 'old ways' of weight loss have prevented people from truly becoming the fat burning machines that they can be.

MYTH 1.

Go into any gym and you will see people slogging it out, doing lots and lots of 'cardio'; repetitive, boring, aerobic-based work, day in and day out. More often than not, for those who continue to flog themselves this way, they very rarely change body shape, nor get the results they are after.

They may shrink and become smaller versions of themselves, but that does not mean to say that they have become fat burning machines; in fact, they can still be carrying worryingly high amounts of fat on their body.

Throughout this book I'll make reference to 'fat loss' but very rarely to 'weight loss.' The reason for this is simple. Weight loss does not take into consideration where that weight has come from; for example, a person may lose weight by losing water, or worse, by losing precious muscle.

LESSON 1
Weight loss is not the same as fat loss!

Fat loss is exactly what it says: removing excessive amounts of fat from your body, while preserving (or improving the amount) lean muscle tissue, so that you may have a better body composition.

Improving the amount of muscle tissue you have on your body is one of the best ways to increase your metabolism and your fat burning potential.

The more muscle you have on your body the more shape you will have, and the better you will look and feel. As you decrease your body fat, and start resistance training you will also experience increases in strength, and an enhanced ability to perform everyday tasks. Plus, you will also look better naked, be able to run after the kids with ease, walk up and down stairs without stopping, and even start participating in activities that you only ever dreamed of taking part in.

Interestingly, muscle tissue is dense and so the more of it you have on your body the heavier you will weigh. On the contrary, fat tissue is not as dense, so when you start adding muscle to your frame you will actually see your weight on the scales *increase;* however, you will also see your body changing shape while the size of your clothing will drop.

These are the desirable fat burning outcomes, so despite what you may have thought up until now, focusing on 'weight loss' and the numbers your scales show you, is *not* the way to gauge your potential fat burning ability.

FACT: MUSCLE OCCUPIES LESS SPACE THAN FAT

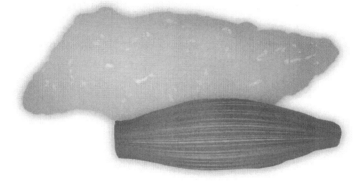

1 kilo of FAT vs 1 kilo of MUSCLE

Now this all said, if you are someone who is grossly obese, just as Kevin was, using scales can be a great measurement tool to help keep you motivated. However, they are just one of many different tools that can be used to monitor progress.

Throughout our journey together, Kev's primary goal was to become a fat burning machine, rather than a weight loss machine.

MYTH 2.

Another common myth is that weight loss can be achieved using a simple equation of monitoring calories in versus calories out.

The body is a complex mechanism and suggesting that all one needs to do is burn more than is ingested is just a small part of the equation (and to be honest, quite outdated).

Effective fat loss is about creating a calorie deficit, while also balancing the complex internal hormones that are responsible for maintaining the proper functioning of the body. If the body's hormonal environment is topsy-turvy, then fat loss is going to be pretty difficult to achieve.

Most weight loss advocates tend to neglect this very important point and so the individual yo-yo cycle of weight loss/weight gain continues.

LESSON 2
Creating the best internal environment for your hormones to do their job properly is actually the key to effective fat loss.

What is a Hormone?
Hormones are chemical messengers that, essentially, control every aspect of our internal functioning. The brain sends these chemical messengers to their specific target cells, with instructions about what to do. They are so potent, in fact, that when we talk about the volume in our body we

refer to them in 'parts per trillion'!

There are certain hormones that greatly affect how your body looks, how much fat is stored (or lost), how much muscle you have, how you perform, your overall energy levels and how hungry you feel. These are the ones that need to be manipulated and taken care of, in order for you to reach your fat burning potential (also, it is these same hormones that are responsible for your overall health).

The hormones that we want to manipulate are cortisol, adrenaline, insulin, glucagon, human growth, testosterone, leptin, and ghrelin. For now we will avoid going into each of the specifics of these hormones, but understand that each one of these hormones and their interactions, have a *direct* effect on your ability to lose fat, put on muscle, stabilise blood sugar levels, regulate and control sleep and stress, and control your hunger.

As you can see, our hormones have the ability to work for us – or in the majority of over-fat people – can actually work against us.

Every element in my Fat Loss Process is designed to optimise your own hormonal profile, so that you can be in the best possible position to turn yourself into a healthy, vibrant, fat burning weapon.

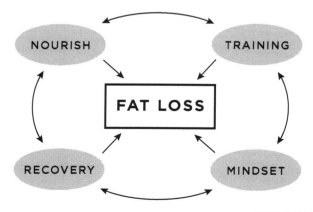

A WORD FROM KEVIN

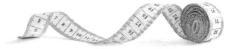

Getting started is harder than it looks and sounds. I, of all people know!

I never wanted to change what I was doing. I was lazy and I was happy to admit it; however, as with all things in life, it starts with just one step.

Congratulations – this book is your first step!

What was my reason for starting?

I had a few reasons (and never wanted to admit to any of them), but I realise now that they were actually always the same.

At the top of my list was my partner Julie. She is my life, my world, and the reason I needed to change. I was stopping her from living her dreams, stopping her from having a life, from travel and from having a relationship with her boyfriend – me.

Another reason was my family. I didn't have a relationship with them because I didn't want to see their faces when they saw how big I had become. I knew they would love me anyway, but I didn't want to deal with that reality.

And of course, another reason was that I was facing death. I was, honestly, just waiting for that big bad thing to happen before I did something to help myself. I was at 268kg, so with 300kg just over the hill, I don't think I was too far away from having to be completely bed-ridden.

With all of this, I needed to act before something really bad happened.

Of course, if you're unlucky enough to have had that 'bad thing' occur, then it's still not too late for you. So long as you have a heartbeat, you have what you need to reverse it and turn it all around.

Meeting Nardia – literally – saved my life. Sure, I was blessed to have a kickstart from The Biggest Loser TV show, but the real key to my success was listening to and learning from her. My journey is far from over, I still have a long way to go, however with my new found knowledge and support from her my future is looking exciting.

She is about to share with you the same things that she shared with me, and all I can say is that it really is kick-arse!

Love,
Big Kev

*'Twenty years from now you will be
more disappointed by the things that
you didn't do than by the ones you did do.
So throw off the bowlines. Sail away from
the safe harbour. Catch the trade winds
in your sails. Explore. Dream. Discover.'*

— MARK TWAIN

THE 10 FAT LOSS PRINCIPLES

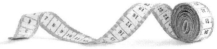

THE 10 FAT LOSS PRINCIPLES ARE:

1. Eat Real Food
2. Eat To Fuel Fat Loss - Starving Yourself Does Not Work
3. Eat Fat, Cut Back On Sugar And Increase Your Protein Intake
4. Drink Yourself Silly
5. Train Smart, Train Hard, Train Often
6. Sleep, Relax and Repair
7. To Change Your Body You Must Change Your Mind
8. Celebrate Your Wins
9. Cultivate The Art Of Mindfulness
10. Take Action!

NOURISH

PRINCIPLE 1:

EAT REAL FOOD

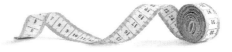

'The food you eat can either be the safest and most powerful form of medicine, or the slowest form of poison.'

— ANN WIGMORE

How your body looks and functions right now, is a direct result of what you have been putting into it. Our body relies on the nutrition that is sourced through food to help it function and perform. If you feed the body poor quality foods then the body itself will be poor in quality and health. This can be recognised in the form of carrying extra fat, muscle aches and pains, poor joint health, a foggy brain and poor digestion.

Your body is an amazing organism. It is constantly growing, adapting and remodeling. It is also the only one you have, so it makes sense to start treating it like an expensive racing car, rather than a garbage disposal!

Every time you eat or drink, the food is broken down into nutrients, and passed into the digestive system where they are then absorbed into the body.

Depending on what you have just eaten will determine where these nutrients go and what the body will use them for. Ultimately, we gain energy from these nutrients, and it is this energy that enables us to live, move and function.

If we ingest an excessive amount of energy, and if that energy comes from a poor source such as processed foods, then we are more likely to end up storing fat, and disrupting the hormones that are designed to keep our body lean.

This is a key point – the quality of the food you eat and the liquids you drink matters.

Eating 'real food' means choosing food that is whole and unprocessed. Foods that are exactly the way Mother Nature intended; not tampered with, not enhanced with additives, preservatives or flavours, not from a packet, just good old-fashioned nutrient-dense foods.

When eating for fat loss, many believe that it is simply a case of reducing your calorie intake; however, time and research has shown that this is not the case. The *quality* of the calorie source is just as important as the quantity that you consume.

Whole foods are those such as vegetables, fruits, some grains, meat, fish, diary, nuts and legumes. These foods contain all the nutrients within the food itself, so when your body breaks them down, they are released in a way that optimises how many nutrients are absorbed and used by the body.

Since the food is organic matter, it is easy for our body to physically break it down and extract the nutrients and energy required for us to function. It is 'easy' on our system (because we have the necessary enzymes needed to break it down within us), and is a natural process. This is why 'whole foods' are considered to be high quality foods.

The same cannot be said for non-real foods such as chocolate, muesli bars, junk food, fish fingers, takeaway meals, frozen pizza and cereal. These are foods that have typically been chemically altered in some way, or contain chemicals, preservatives, additives, flavours, colours, trans-fats, high fructose corn syrups or the like. As a result, they are often more challenging for the body to break down and will result in a very different effect on your physiology than 'whole' foods from quality sources. These foods are considered poor quality foods.

The greater the amount of poor quality foods that you consume, the more difficult it becomes for your body to stay lean and healthy. What's more, the effects of the chemicals become cumulative. Over time, these compounds can be interpreted as 'toxic' within the body, and end up being stored on the body, simply because they cannot be excreted. This is usually because large amounts of these foods can start to challenge the liver, which is the organ responsible for detoxifying the body.

Interestingly, there is only one place in the body that can store toxins, and that is in our fat cells.

If there is an overload of toxins that the body cannot cope with it *will* create more fat stores to cope with the demand. These added compounds also wreak havoc on the hormonal system by interfering with the natural release of certain hormones. These toxins have the ability to stimulate release of hormones, inhibit release of hormones or mimic certain hormones, all of which disrupts the body's natural processes. As a result fat loss is hindered and your overall health is jeopardised.

WHAT ABOUT 'DIET' PRODUCTS?

Diet products such as artificial sweeteners, diet fizzy drinks, diet jellies and lollies fall into the category of non-real foods. As such they should be considered detrimental to your fat loss goal and should not be consumed.

Most of them are created with synthetic chemicals and, oddly enough, can actually lead to *more* fat gain. Non-caloric artificial sweeteners such as aspartame and saccharine have been shown to increase appetite by interfering with the body's appetite control system, leading to an overall increase in calorie consumption. The actual sweetness of these chemicals is also responsible for promoting more cravings of sweet food. So even though it seems that you are doing yourself a favour by consuming them, you are actually potentially adding more stress to your system.

Many people make the mistake of pursuing fat loss at the expense of their health. They may reduce their overall calorie intake, train poorly or consume loads of diet products thinking that they are doing the right thing. Whilst they may seem to achieve some short term gains, it is in actual fact, setting them up for failure in the long term.

Effective long term fat loss occurs when you keep your body healthy. High quality 'real foods', not only provides the body with energy, but it also helps nurture it both now and in the future. The vitamins, minerals and antioxidants found in real foods mean you are going to experience fat loss, but in addition you'll also see and feel improvements in your general health and wellbeing.

HOW TO TELL THE DIFFERENCE BETWEEN A REAL FOOD AND A NON-REAL FOOD

In a supermarket, it can often be confusing to work out what foods are more 'real' than others. If it is not in a package, then it is safe to assume that it is a fresh food item.

Of course, sometimes it is necessary to purchase foods that come in a package. In this instance, a simple way to work out if it is a good choice is to look at the food label. If the ingredients list is made up of a long list of numbers and words that you cannot pronounce on the back, then do not purchase it. More often than not, the more numbers and complicated words there are, the more synthesised (or chemically affected) it is, and it is best to be avoided.

You also want to pay attention to the order of the ingredients that are listed. This is because, normally, the largest contained ingredient is listed first, so you should always look to ensure that the ingredients list reflects the product you are buying. For example, when I took a look at a popular chocolate flavoured milk drink, I found 'cocoa' listed fifth on the ingredient list after milk, cream, sugar, and high fructose corn syrup!

A great tip for locating real foods is to avoid the supermarket aisles in the middle of the store, and head towards the more open spaced parts of your supermarket, which is typically where you'll find fresh fruit, vegetables and meats. Most packaged, 'fake' foods tend to be located on the shelves in those middle aisles.

Another great place to shop for real food is your local farmers' markets. Not only is the produce local and fresh, it can sometimes even be a bit cheaper. Despite what many think, eating fresh, quality food is no more expensive than supermarket food.

KEY POINTS

1. Eat real food.
2. Avoid packaged, fake, non-foods (this includes liquids).
3. The quality of the food is just as important as the amount of food being eaten.
4. Eat for both fat loss and good health.
5. If a food label has loads of numbers on it or words you cannot pronounce then avoid it!

PRINCIPLE 2:

EAT TO FUEL FAT LOSS — STARVING DOES NOT WORK!

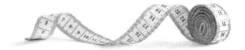

I love this point because, let's face it, eating is something that brings us so much joy. It is ritualistic and often a very social affair. Unfortunately, when it comes to fat loss it is assumed that the only way to get results is by 'cutting calories' and becoming super rigid with low calorie diets. Not only is this boring and depressing, it is also a surefire way to encourage binge eating at a later stage.

Whenever you go on a 'diet' to lose fat, you are essentially putting yourself on a restricted plan. This 'restriction' alone, sets up a negative environment and mindset, in which you are destined to fail. Diets assume that you are either 'on' or 'off' with no allowance for mood, variability, energy levels or life!

People who are always dieting are the ones who have that mindset of 'I can't', 'I can't have this, or I can't have that', and end up spending so much time and energy focusing on the things that they 'cant' have that they end up breaking and binging on the forbidden 'fruit' with vengeance. This is particularly true for those on super low calorie diets (e.g., the ones below 1,200 calories, which should actually never be used unless under medical supervision).

From the outset, low calorie diets are setting you up for failure. Yes, they may seem appealing because weight loss results are produced quite quickly, but this is only a short-term result, not a long term one.

Two reasons why low calories diets don't work is because, as I mentioned earlier, the 'weight loss' is rather indiscriminate, and most likely that rapid weight loss is coming from precious muscle, rather than from fat stores. I've also alluded to the fact that losing muscle interferes with the body's metabolism (a key to ongoing fat loss). Two, the body has a strong evolutionary survival mechanism which, when starved of calories, tends to kick in. Here, the appetite becomes reduced, the hormones are interfered with, and psychological impacts occur. Low calorie diets will, more often than not, result in fat gains and health issues down the track.

To be successful with your fat loss it is important to adopt a new lifestyle as opposed to a diet. Eating for fat loss and good health is a way of life – not something that you are temporarily 'on' or 'off'.

As you learn more about good nutrition, health and how your body responds to food you will find the best eating style for you – one that allows you the flexibility to eat when you want, and what you want. By this I mean, when you adopt a new way of healthy eating you will no longer *want* to eat crap food – I guarantee it. You will choose to eat healthy because you'll enjoy it – trust me on this! However, I want to make something very clear; eating lots of high quality food is not giving you the green light to go ahead and over-indulge. You still need to be mindful of what you are eating. You just don't need to be ruled by it.

It is also important to understand that while I do not recommend rigid calorie counting (as this can become highly restrictive), you do need to realise that a calorie has a consequence.

If you overeat and ingest a lot of calories, above and beyond your body's need, you will gain weight. And this is particularly true if these calories are coming from a poor source. However, the same can be said if you over-consume a lot of so-called 'good foods' like gluten-free cookies, 'health' bars, 'Paleo' desserts and so forth. Constant over-consumption of calories will lead to a change in body composition – and not for the better.

To reiterate an earlier point, not all calorie sources are created equal, and depending on what the sources are, will determine how it is used in your body. For example, eating 2,000 calories of greens vegetables, lean meats and nuts will not yield the same result as eating 2,000 calories of chocolate. A daily intake of calories that come from food sources such as cornflakes, skim milk, bread, deli meats, pasta, takeaways, biscuits, fizzy drinks or desserts will, over time lead to fat gains. These particular foods are all examples of 'energy-dense, nutrient-sparse' foods because they contain large amounts of energy with very little nutritional benefits. Not only will this type of eating wreak havoc on your appearance, it will also be detrimental to your health.

By focusing on ingesting foods that are nutrient-rich, and

energy-light, such as vegetables, salads, lean meats (e.g., chicken and beef) fish, nuts and full-fat probiotic yoghurt you will provide your body with huge nutritional benefits, while also staying satisfied and full. The calories that are sourced from these high quality foods will have a positive effect on your hormones, your overall health and will, ultimately, lead to fat loss (so long as they are not over-consumed).

The next focus, after including more great quality food, is to work on portion size. In general, people overestimate the amount of 'good' food they eat and underestimate the amount of 'bad' food they eat.

GETTING THE SIZE RIGHT

There are a few different methods for working out servings sizes or portion control, with the two most popular being the 'measuring' method and the second being the 'guesstimated palm-size' method.

Both are effective, and I suggest that you play around with which method works best for you. Remember, this is about you gaining enough information so that you can make educated decisions regarding your food choices.

In the 'measuring' method, every food item is weighed or measured so that you can visually learn what a serving size is. This is a great tool to use in the initial stages because it helps you gain an appreciation for the right sizes. I recall the first time I ever measured my serving size of vegetables and realised that I was eating way below the recommendation, even though I thought I was eating the right amount.

Measuring foods is not likely to become a long term

solution, because after just a few weeks you'll have a very good understanding of what the right serving size actually is. This leads you, naturally, to the 'guesstimated palm-size' method.

The best portable measuring tools that you have are, literally, your hands. This is because the size of your hands is proportionate to your body, making it a very useful tool.

Quite simply:
- the palm of your hand (the width and thickness) equates to a serving size of protein
- a closed fist equates to a serving size of vegetables (the greens ones)
- a cupped hand equates to a serving size of a carbohydrate portion (such as fruit, rice, quinoa and starchy vegetables such as a sweet potato)
- the thumb length and thickness equates to a portion of fat.

The palm-size method is particularly useful when trying to work out what a plate of food should look like.

When serving up food on a plate, to help get your portions right simply break your plate up into sections:

- half the plate should be filled with non-starchy vegetables, like greens
- a quarter of the plate should have a lean protein source
- the other quarter should have a carbohydrate such as sweet potato, quinoa, legumes or rice
- while fats, like dressing or butter, can be added on top.

YOUR PLATE BREAKDOWN

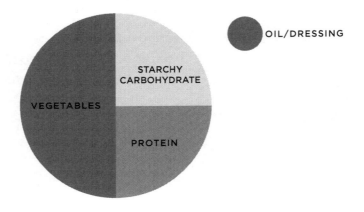

KEY POINTS

1. Eat lots of quality food – foods that contain lots of nutrients without a lot of energy.
2. Not all sources of calories are created equal – some are better than others.
3. Get your portions under control by either measuring your food, or guesstimating the portions by using the palm-size method.
4. Build your plate of food the same way every time.

PRINCIPLE 3:

EAT FAT, CUT BACK ON SUGAR AND INCREASE YOUR PROTEIN INTAKE

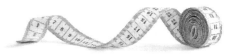

EAT FAT

Somebody once told me that they believed that ingested dietary fat turns to fat and, therefore, overweight people shouldn't eat fat. It was believed that overweight people should stick to low fat options and limit the amount of fat they consume. Have you heard this? If so, you are not alone. Since the 1980s when there was a strong push towards a low fat way of eating, there has been a massive 'fat shaming', 'fat scared' mentality which, unfortunately, has been at the detriment of a lot of waistlines (and health).

The truth is, the above notion is absolute hogwash. If it

were true, then every time someone ate protein it would instantly turn to muscle – and while the gym junkies would be loving it, it's just not possible.

Fat is not the enemy. It is not as scary or as damaging as previously thought, and it is only in recent times that people are truly understanding the importance of *quality* fat for health and – in fact – fat loss.

In our body there are two types of different fats: white adipose tissue and brown adipose tissue. The fat that layers our body and, in circumstances where there is too much, the stuff that hangs over our belts is called 'subcutaneous fat'. This fat is designed to keep us warm, acts as a storage unit for energy, and offers protection for our body. Fat that builds up internally around organs is called 'visceral fat', and while it is also designed as a protective mechanism for our organs, when there is too much of it, it becomes a risk factor for heart disease, hypertension and diabetes. Both subcutaneous and visceral fat are white adipose tissue.

Fat constituents are also found in other areas of the body, such as the brain and the layers of your cells.

Currently there is new research emerging exploring the role of brown adipose tissue. We have high levels of brown fat when we are a baby and infant, and its role is to help with heat production. As we age we tend to lose this adipose tissue so, comparatively, as adults we have a lot less brown fat than we do white fat. The exciting thing is that scientists have identified that brown adipose tissue is metabolically active, which means it has the potential to use calories to produce heat. Results are still preliminary but it seems that exposure to cold and training are good ways to increase the amount of brown fat in the body, and it is being investigated further as another potential way to combat obesity.

Our brain, which is made up of fat and water, needs certain good fats (derived from dietary fat) in order to function. Without these good fats in our diets our brain cannot assemble the necessary building blocks that are needed for optimal brain health and brain function. In other words, if the brain is not getting the good stuff then you are likely to suffer from cloudy thinking, decreased cognitive performance, and are more likely to suffer from mental health issues such as depression and anxiety (this of course can also contribute to emotional eating, and negative thought processes through changes in brain chemistry).

Most of the food we eat can be categorised into one of three categories:

- fats
- carbohydrates
- protein

Collectively these are known as macronutrients, as the bulk of our diets come from these sources.

Vitamins, minerals and antioxidants fall into the category of micronutrients. Although we do not need large amounts of micronutrients, they are very important for overall functioning of our internal system.

In order to achieve long-term fat loss, it is important that your macronutrients come from quality sources. This is where fat shaming went wrong. Rather than recommending that all sources of fats be eliminated from our diet, what should have occurred is that people should have been encouraged to eliminate the poor quality sources of fats. What actually occurred was that eating guidelines began to promote a 'low-fat' ideal which, unfortunately, led to a 'high-carb' (and high sugar) style of eating, and that turned out to be even more damaging to people's physiques and overall health.

When it comes to fat, we actually need to source two particular types of fatty acids from our diet, because our body is unable to make them. These fats are called 'essential fatty acids'. You may have heard of them: omega 3s and omega 6s. The other important fatty acid is omega 9, but this is not considered essential, because your body can actually produce it if there is an adequate supply of both omega 3s and 6s.

Omega fats are essential for your overall health and body composition, and while one is not better than the other, if there is an imbalance between them, then poor health will result.

Interestingly, the health conditions that can occur are due to an increase in systemic inflammation. Omega 3s are considered to be anti-inflammatory in nature, whereas omega 6 are said to be pro-flammatory (as an aside it is now widely recognised that chronic inflammation is a pre-cursor to many diseases such as Alzheimer's Disease, heart disease, arthritis and kidney failure).

It is largely agreed that the ratio of omega 6s to omega 3s should lie between 2:1 and 5:1. Unfortunately, it has been estimated that the ratio in the western world is more like 15:1! The reason for this huge discrepancy is due to the large amounts of sugary, processed foods that are consumed, and a concurrent lack in consumption of foods rich in omega 3s.

The major food culprits that are driving our omega 6s to dangerous levels are those containing cheaply manufactured seed oils. These include generic vegetable oils, canola, rice bran, peanut, sesame, corn (maize), cottonseed, sunflower, soybean, grapeseed and safflower oils. When you look at the ingredients list of any packaged food, it is highly likely that you will see one or more of these on the label.

Other poor quality fats such as trans-fats (trans-fatty acids) or partially hydrogenated fats, are artificial fats that have been chemically altered to improve the overall consistency and texture of a product. For years they have been used in commercially baked products such as donuts, biscuits, crackers, fried foods, fast food chains and margarines. The major detrimental effect that trans-fats have on the body is that they increase the amount of 'bad' cholesterol, and decrease the amount of 'good' cholesterol. This leads to a substantial increase in risk for heart disease and certain types of cancer.

Seed oils, and artificial oils are toxic for your body and should be avoided.

By crowding out the poor quality foods with good quality foods the ratio of omega 6s to omega 3s can be restored, and with it, all the benefits of improved health.

Your goal should be to consume quality sources of fats, such as organic butter, ghee, coconut oil, coconut butter, nuts, avocado, fish, olive oil and lean meats. Not only will your tastebuds thank you but so, too, will your body.

Now you may be thinking 'hang on a minute, isn't fat really high in calories? Didn't you say to be mindful of this?' The answer to both would be 'yes' – fats are high in calories and they do pack an 'energy punch', which is why it is necessary to be mindful of how much you eat. Again, just because I am advising including fats into your daily eating, it is not a green light to over-indulge on them. Portion control is very important. Normally when we talk about portion sizes for fats we use small measurements such as a teaspoon or tablespoon at a time (or a thumb's worth) – never huge quantities.

Think of your fats like this: a little amount, often, goes a long way.

CUT BACK ON SUGAR

Most of the sugar that is eaten is not from you sprinkling extra onto your cereal, or adding it to your coffee. Instead, it is already included in your food items by the manufacturers.

It has been estimated that the average Australian consumes around 42kg of sugar per year, which equates to about 28 teaspoons per day. Of course, this is just an estimate, and it can be assumed that if a diet is high in processed, packaged food and soft drinks, and low in good quality fresh ingredients that this number could be even higher.

Excessive amounts of sugar in the diet have been linked to not only fat gain and diabetes, but also inflammatory diseases, much like poor quality fats.

Sugar per se is not the devil, but the mass overconsumption of it and the lack of quality nutrients eaten as a result, is. Similar to the notion of fat sources, the type of sugar being consumed can also be beneficial or harmful.

All carbohydrates break down to form sugar molecules, with the simplest being glucose. This is what we know as 'sugar'. There are a many different types of carbohydrates and they can be classified as either a 'simple carbohydrate' or a 'complex carbohydrate' (this is determined by their chemical structure). In general its structural classification will determine how quickly the glucose enters our blood stream.

Most people know that foods like bread, rice, pasta and grains are carbohydrates, but so too are vegetables, fruit, and legumes. This means that a sweet potato, when digested and broken down into its smallest molecules, will become sugar and provide the blood stream with glucose. But so too will an apple, a plate of beans or a bag of lollies. However, all these foods will have a very different impact on your hormonal system and, therefore, your body.

The high quality sources of carbohydrates – and the ones that you want to base a high portion of your daily intake on – are those that contain loads of fibre, and that release glucose into the blood stream slowly. Vegetables, whole grains, and legumes are good examples of this. One of the fundamental elements in fuelling fat loss is keeping the body's blood sugar levels relatively stable.

Poor quality carbohydrates, such as highly refined and processed foods, should be avoided and include white breads, rice, pasta, baked goods, confectionary, commercial sauces and non-cultured yoghurts containing high levels of sugar. This is because, when ingested these foods release glucose into the blood stream very quickly. When the body senses an increase in blood sugar levels it releases the hormone 'insulin' to encourage the blood glucose to move into the cells (muscle and liver), storing it as energy. In most circumstances this process works well, but when a diet is predominantly based on simple, highly refined carbohydrates it wrecks havoc on the hormonal system.

The internal workings of the body are impressive; it can withstand a multitude of stressors – whether they be nutritional, chemical or psychological. But if, over time, they are not supported then the inner workings will start to break down.

Typically a blood sugar 'high' is accompanied with a blood sugar 'low', which is normally followed up by an increase in hunger and the need to eat again. You can see this reaction quite clearly in children – when they have had a load of lollies (simple sugar), they get a rush of energy, which is usually followed by a massive crash or come down, and they may get grumpy and tired as a result. As adults we do the same thing, however at that point of 'come down' we may also experience brain fog, the inability to concentrate and light-headedness. At this point, most adults will reach for something to eat again to provide them with some more energy. Unfortunately, if the 'go-to' food is another simple, refined carbohydrate then another 'high-low' cycle will result. If this style of eating is repeated over a long period of time then the sensitivity of the hormone insulin will decrease and more and more blood glucose will be required in order for insulin to encourage glucose into the cells. What you end up with is high blood glucose and insulin resistance that will, if not treated, lead to type 2 diabetes.

In days gone by type 2 diabetes was also called 'adult onset diabetes', because it was most common in adults. Today, however, more and more children are experiencing type 2 diabetes.

As a result, it has recently been named the 'lifestyle' disease and has been connected with health conditions such as increased obesity, blood pressure and high cholesterol. Apart from some genetic predisposition, most of the risk factors for type 2 diabetes are lifestyle based; in other words, nutrition and training play a huge role in both the development and treatment of this disease. If there is a lack of good quality nutrient-rich, energy-sparse foods in conjunction with a sedentary lifestyle, then the risk for type 2 diabetes increases.

I wont go into too much detail here about children, but

it is an issue that needs to be addressed. Children and adolescents should not be exhibiting adult-type diseases, but because of our current eating habits and sedentary lifestyles it is happening more and more. The physical and psychological stress that is being placed on overweight children is not acceptable, and it certainly does not bode well for our future generations. Typically, an over-fat child will have over-fat parents because children model behaviour from their parents. By embarking on this Fat Loss Process, not only will you be improving your health and the way you look and feel, but if you have children then you can also influence their future, as well as others around you.

When food manufacturers learned that they could create cheap oils and artificial fats such as trans-fats, they also worked out they could do the same with sugar. One of the most toxic artificial sugars to date is high fructose corn syrup (HFCS), a corn-based sweetener that also goes by the name of high fructose maize syrup. HFCS is found in most processed, poor quality food products such as fizzy drinks, packaged foods, juices, sauces and syrups. It is used because it is cheaper than standard cane sugar, and it is actually sweeter in taste. HFCS should not be confused with 'fructose', which is a naturally occurring sugar found in most plants (e.g., fruit, and vegetables).

Natural fructose is found in nutrient-dense whole foods that also contain fibre. For example, in fruit and vegetables the naturally occurring sugars are wrapped up with all the fibre and so have a different affect on the body when digested and absorbed than HFCS. Apart from the fibre, fruit and vegetables also provide a host of other goodies such as essential vitamins, minerals, phytonutrients and antioxidants. Eating fruit and vegetables on a daily basis *will* promote good health and fat loss.

The metabolism of HFCS is very different from natural sugar, and large consumption of this artificial substance has been linked to non-alcoholic liver disease, increased appetite, obesity and inflammation.

Remember, sugar can also sneak its way onto food labels, disguised as other words. Keep an eye out for words such as: 'nectars', 'syrups', 'corn syrups', 'juice', 'cane crystals', 'cane juice crystals', 'sweeteners', 'maltodextrin', 'treacle' and any words that end in 'ose'. This may seem like an extensive list, but if you are choosing foods that are real, whole foods you won't have to worry too much. After all, most real foods don't come packaged with an ingredients list!

In a promising move, the Australian government is now recognising the potential health risk of sugar consumption and in it's newly released Australian Dietary Guidelines has recommended 'limited' amounts of food that contain added sugar.

INCREASE YOUR PROTEIN INTAKE

For a long time protein has been synonymous with bodybuilders wanting to increase the amount of lean muscle in their body in order to look bigger. They do this by manipulating their training and by consuming large amounts of protein such as meat, eggs, nuts and protein powders.

Now, you may not want to look like Arnold Schwarzenegger at the peak of his bodybuilding career, but since fat loss is the goal, then increasing the amount of quality protein in your diet is a must. Protein is necessary for virtually every cellular function in our body. At a metabolic level protein is crucial, however it is also crucial for the development of our muscles.

Developing a good body composition is the aim of this Fat Loss Process, and that requires encouraging fat loss while also improving the amount of lean muscle in the body. Besides an effective training program this can be achieved by consuming good quality sources of protein.

Often, protein is the most under-eaten of all macronutrients. When ingested, protein is broken into it's smallest molecules – amino acids. These amino acids form the building blocks of everything in our body and can be further broken into two types: essential amino acids and non-essential amino acids. As the names suggest, the essential ones are the ones that the body cannot make and, therefore, relies solely on food sources for provision.

One of the advantages of eating more protein is that it improves satiety, and helps regulate appetite. Just like fat, ingesting protein will leave you feeling more full, satisfied for longer and less likely to snack on poor quality foods. It will also have a positive effect on your blood sugar levels, particularly if the protein comes from an animal source.

All quality animal sources of protein (such as chicken, fish, beef, turkey, kangaroo, eggs, cheese and cultured yoghurt) are considered 'complete' protein sources as they contain all the essential amino acids.

Protein that comes from plant sources (such as legumes, nuts, tofu, tempeh, edamame, seeds and nuts) are considered 'incomplete' as they only contain certain amino acids. Even though it may seem that gaining protein from animal sources alone would be ideal, it is important to include some plant sources.

There are some meat sources that should be avoided due to high levels of salt, preservatives and other nasties. These include salami, packaged meats like ham, some bacon (nitrous free bacon is okay), sausages, frozen meats like chicken nuggets, fish fingers and pies.

REQUIRED DAILY SERVINGS

	Carbo-hydrates (vegeta-bles)	Carbo-hydrates (starchy and fruit)	Protein	Fat	Dairy*
M	4-5	2-3	4-5	3-4	1-2
F	2-3	1-2	3-4	2-3	1-2

Dairy may or may not be tolerated therefore may be omitted. However, good quality fats such as grass-fed butter and hard cheese eg. gouda or parmesan are often better tolerated and therefore may be included.

Please also see Appendices for examples of serving sizes for each food group.

KEY POINTS

1. Eat more quality fats: butter, ghee, coconut oil, olive oil; avoid trans-fat, vegetable oils and hydrogenated fats.
2. Avoid sugar, especially the fake kinds.
3. Eat quality protein with every meal.

THERE IS NO SUCH THING AS FALLING OFF THE WAGON

According to the State Government of Victoria 'Australians spend up to one million dollars a day on fad diets that have little effect on their weight loss.'

How many times have you tried to 'diet?'

Did it work?

Like many, it may have produced certain results at the time, however, if you have not been able to sustain those results, then it can be considered as being very unsuccessful.

In these modern times, the word 'diet' is associated with negative, restrictive protocols and, often, people who diet are either 'on' or 'off' one at any point in time. This is a stark contrast to the original meaning, which comes from the Greek word 'diata' or 'dieta', meaning 'a way of life, mode of living.'

We need to move back towards the original meaning, to focus our mindset on creating a healthy relationship with food and to formulate healthy food habits that create a positive 'way of life' and 'mode of living'.

In order to be successful with your fat loss you must understand that you are not 'on' or 'off' a diet. Instead, you are simply creating a new eating lifestyle. A lifestyle that allows you the flexibility to eat a wide range of foods without restricting or limiting you, and one that caters for fluctuations in your hunger, environment, mood and energy levels. It is possible to get results and remain healthy while eating tasty, interesting and non-restrictive foods.

Instead of thinking about either being 'on' or 'off' a diet, consider yourself as fluctuating. There are some days where you may be extra hungry, and there are other days where your appetite is less; this is completely normal and learning how to eat for those days is important. If you are genuinely hungry then eat more and refuel yourself as required. If your appetite has diminished then, simply, don't eat as much.

We are not designed to eat the same amount of food at a set time, every day of every week. While there are certainly predictable rhythms that our body is accustomed to, learning to listen to your body, and what it is telling you is a crucial part of achieving and maintaining long term fat loss.

The more in-tune you are with your body and how it feels at any given moment, the better you will be at making the adjustments necessary to achieve the results you desire.

Being attuned with your body will also help you in your quest to form healthy relationships with food. Now, 'having a relationship with food' might seem like an odd concept, but if you think about it how you use food, and why you eat is often intertwined with your emotions. Apart from when there are legitimate physical food cravings, a lot of the time we actually use food to make us feel a certain way.

When you eat, do you ever think things such as:

- 'I can't eat that because it's bad'
- 'I can treat myself to that because I've been so good lately'.

Many of us have an internal dialogue like this, when it comes to eating, and we are constantly giving food a label of 'good' or 'bad'. As a result, this label can become a judgment upon ourselves. For example, if a perceived 'good' food is eaten, then we feel like we are a 'good', person. Similarly, if a 'bad' food is eaten, then we feel a sense of shame and guilt.

As you can see, food can sometimes be directly tied into how we feel about ourselves.

Judging yourself based on the food you eat is not conducive to helping you lose fat. In fact, the more you judge yourself, the more likely you are to remain trapped in a negative mindset, which will never be useful in helping you achieve your fat loss goals.

To improve this unhealthy relationship, you should start to view food as either being 'nurturing' or 'less nurturing', with the aim to eat more foods that fall into the 'nurturing' category. By following the advice in the previous pages about eating real, wholesome foods, you will – by default – be consuming nurturing foods.

KNOW THE DIFFERENCE BETWEEN PHYSICAL HUNGER AND EMOTIONAL HUNGER

In life there are many things that we hunger for. Everyday we are faced with physical hunger, the type that is accelerated by our body's internal environment to drive us to physically eat and drink, but this is often overridden by another type of hunger – emotional hunger. In other words, there is a difference between true hunger and eating emotionally.

Food, with all of its different tastes, textures and smells, is to be enjoyed, and the physical act of eating is a wonderful thing. So, on the odd occasion it is completely normal to want to use food as a small reward for a job well done. However, the problem arises when reaching for food becomes the coping mechanism for all your emotions.

Knowing the difference between physical and emotional

hunger is a big step towards helping you to understand and recognise the 'why' behind your eating.

Many different feelings trigger emotional eating, such as being stressed, tired, sad, happy, depressed or lonely; and the type of emotion you are feeling may well determine what type of food you crave.

To understand the difference between physical hunger and emotional hunger you need to first identify the onset. When you are physically hungry, there is a gradual onset and it starts with a slight rumbling of the tummy, which if left, turns into a growling and a gnawing at the stomach. The hunger can be felt in the stomach area, and can instantly be satisfied by eating something. When you are truly physically hungry, lots of different types of food options will sound appealing (even vegetables!).

On the other hand, if an emotional hunger is being experienced there will be a craving towards specific foods. Normally these foods include things such as pizza, burgers, chocolate, ice cream, alcohol and crisps, and no matter how much is consumed there is still a feeling of dissatisfaction. This can lead to what I call 'frenzied eating' or 'bingeing,' where the entire act of indulging becomes a mindless process.

If you've ever felt bored, upset, angry or sad then you may have experienced this yourself. Not surprisingly, after one of these frenzies it is easy to feel worse than beforehand, especially if the binge is followed by a sense of guilt or shame, which often further perpetuates the initial emotional state.

Medicating yourself with food to try and numb yourself from your emotions should never be the answer. This process will lead to fat gains but will also create a negative relationship with food, where food becomes your 'frenemy'. It comforts you, yet only causes damage to your health and wellbeing in the long run.

Understanding that you may be eating due to emotional reasons will open your mind to identifying what is really troubling you, and provides the opportunity to develop a non-food strategy to deal with your emotional needs. By acknowledging the cravings, you can tame them without giving into them.

NON-FOOD STRATEGIES TO DEAL WITH EMOTIONS

If you have identified that you are, in fact, emotionally eating, the first thing you should do is put distance between the emotion and your automated reaction to reach for food. It is important to note that there is a clear distinction between the definition of 'overeating', and 'eating emotionally'.

It is also important to note that there are clinically diagnosed conditions such as 'Binge Eating Disorder' and 'Compulsive Eating Disorder'. If you feel you have either of these conditions or if you wish to find out more about them, then you should consult a professional who specialises in this area. What I'm providing solutions for are those of us who, typically speaking, use food as a 'go-to' strategy for solving an emotional problem. For these people, placing distance between the emotion and the habit of eating can be effective, and involves interrupting your usual thought patterns to introduce a new approach.

For instance, you can try distracting yourself by going for a walk, training, immersing yourself in tasks, calling a friend, putting on music, meditating, or doing something creative.

Another method is to try visualising different images that are not associated with food, such as flowers, people and objects. Or you could try reciting poetry, stories or singing a song. It is also possible to try and 'wait out the craving' by saying something like 'If, in 15 minutes, I am still wanting X, Y, Z and I am truly hungry then I will allow myself to eat X, Y, Z'.

Meanwhile, as you distance yourself from the food, you need to address the emotional reason behind the craving. Ask yourself these types of questions:

- 'What am I really feeling? Am I sad, angry, depressed, lonely or bored?'
- 'Why am I feeling this way?'
- 'If I eat X, Y, Z am I actually going to feel better? Will this food solve my emotional problem?
- 'How can I really solve these emotional feelings? Do I need to seek professional help, talk to friends or family, join a community or club, or find a new job? How can I add more joy into my life?'

By becoming more aware of your feelings and emotions, you can start to overcome underlying issues that are currently preventing your fat loss success.

KEY POINTS

1. Become in-tune with your body.
2. Understand the difference between real hunger and emotional hunger.
3. If you experience an emotional craving, create distance between the emotion and the action of eating.

THE 'METABOLISM' TRUTH BOMB

The most ideal way of eating throughout any one day is a hotly contested issue among dietitians, nutritionists, health professionals and personal trainers.

The most popular methodologies include:

- eating six times a day (called the 'Frequent Feeding Model', using three main meals interspersed with three snacks)
- eating three square meals per day
- constant grazing all day.

While each method has valid arguments, advocates for the six meals per day and grazing methods use the argument that the metabolism needs to be 'stoked' like a fire, in order to keep it running so that the body is in peak physiological position to burn body fat.

The three meals per day advocates suggest that by sticking to three square meals a day, less calories will be consumed overall, therefore providing a better solution for fat loss.

So what is the correct way to consume your meals? The answer is pretty simple – whichever one suits you best! In order to understand that answer, let me explain metabolism in a little more detail.

'Metabolism' is probably one of the misused words in the weight loss and fitness industries. Too often people have blamed their 'slow metabolism' for their less than ideal body shape. While it is certainly true that in some medical circumstances a slow metabolism can be blamed for an increase in weight, it is not the norm.

Your metabolism is the rate at which your body burns calories in a day – the amount needed in order for you to function. If you were to lie in bed all day (and thus, not expending any energy) this would be considered your Basal Metabolic Rate (BMR), or the amount of calories needed at rest. Interestingly, the bigger someone is the more likely that his or her BMR is higher! Not slow, as most may assume. This is because the more weight on a body, the more energy is required to function.

This also explains why it is easier, in a sense, for a much bigger person to lose weight quickly through simple methods of changing eating habits – it's because their metabolism is running higher. Of course, this only works in the short term and after a while the weight loss will slow down. Kev was a classic example of this. He was able to shred 13kg in the first few weeks of his new eating plan, simply by cutting out all the fizzy drinks.

But here is the double-edged sword: the more weight that is lost (and more so if a lot of muscle tissue is lost), the less calories that person will require to function, meaning they should actually eat less. Therefore, the metabolism needs to somehow be increased, in order to keep the "calorie-burning fire" going.

Enter the food and metabolism myth
Multi-billion dollar weight loss companies pride themselves on products that claim to 'boost the metabolism' to help 'burn more fat!' The fact is, these claims are misleading.

Neither food nor supplements have a large affect on metabolism. For sure, the physical act of digesting food and distributing the nutrients requires energy, but for the most part it is negligible.

Instead, your age, gender and genetics play a role in determining your metabolism, with the most influential factor being the amount of lean muscle tissue you have on your body. Lean muscle tissue is metabolically active, meaning that it will burn calories at rest – and a lot more calories than fat tissue will!

Quality strength training will improve and preserve the amount of lean muscle tissue you have, therefore, positively affecting your BMR. This is why weight training is a critical component when seeking long term fat loss.

Based on this information you can see that your metabolism will not become super-slow if you choose to only eat three times in a day; and nor will it go into hyper-drive if you choose to eat more regularly.

When deciding the best method and frequency to consume your nutrients, there are some considerations to take into account. Factors such as your work, home schedule, and natural hunger levels will contribute to identifying which eating plan will best suit you.

The key is to choose the method that is easy to stick with. In some circumstances people work in jobs that only allow for a set number of breaks; therefore, it may suit them to choose the three square meals a day regime. Starting the day with a hearty breakfast will be enough to tie them over until lunchtime, and then a good solid lunch will get them through to dinnertime.

Other people will be in a position that allows more flexibility for snacking between meals.

As I mentioned, there is no right or wrong here. It's a case of doing what works the best for you. And it might be a case of trying a few different ways until you find the one that feels right. Now this is, of course, all on the proviso that you are consuming only nutrient-dense foods, are maintaining stable energy levels throughout the day and are without emotional food cravings.

Despite the lack of agreement among professionals over the ideal daily meal distribution, the one meal that is definitely agreed on is the one consumed after a workout. I will delve into this later on in the book, but for now just know that eating a meal immediately post-training is critical for the repair of your body and in order to achieve fat loss.

Remember this Fat Loss Process is about you becoming the expert in you. Honing into the elements that work best for you is what will ensure long-term success. So, choose the style of meal timing that will enable you to successfully stick to a good healthy eating routine.

PRINCIPLE 4:

DRINK YOURSELF SILLY

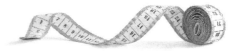

As a kid I was often told to drink more water. Not exactly what a child wants to hear because back then, to me, water was tasteless and boring. Fast-forward to today and I cannot get enough of it.

Around 60 per cent of our body is water, so without it we would die. If ever stranded on an island you could survive for a couple of weeks without food by living off the reserves of fat and muscle in your body; however, you would not be able to survive more than three to five days without water to drink. Water is our life source.

Virtually every metabolic process in our body requires water; from temperature regulation, to lubrication, to digestion and for forming the basis of our blood. Since we cannot store water we need to consume it on daily basis. For most, depending on your size, around two to three litres per day is required (which can be sourced from the foods you eat and liquids you drink).

To say that water consumption is important, is an understatement. Yet many of us go through our days in a state of dehydration. This is amplified if your diet is high in processed foods and liquids, and absent of quality real foods (particularly vegetables) and water.

It actually does not take much for the body to become slightly dehydrated; in fact a two per cent decrease in hydration can have large negative effects, such as headaches, dizziness, brain fog, dry mouth and thirst.

In the short term, rehydrating can solve this dehydration; however, chronic low levels of dehydration can cause the body more serious problems. Being in a chronic state of dehydration can cause weakening of the cellular environment of the body, which can lead to a variety of other problems. When this is compounded with poor nutrition, obesity and stress, the effects are far more serious.

The interesting thing about chronic dehydration is that eventually the body accepts the state as the new 'normal' and, as such, the thirst response becomes blunted. So, paradoxically the longer you are in a state of dehydration the less likely you are to have thirst as an indicator. Other symptoms will occur but they are far subtler than the obvious dry mouth and thirst.

WATER FOR FAT LOSS

From a fat loss perspective, drinking loads of water is crucial. Of particular importance to the Fat Loss Process is the way the body metabolises fat; and how well fat is metabolised is determined by the health of your liver.

The liver is an incredible organ that is responsible for many different functions in the body that relate to detoxification, production of bile, breakdown of fats, and immunity (to name only a few). Because the liver is involved with so many different processes in the body we do rely heavily on its ability to keep us functioning.

The liver will break fats down into its simplest forms, which can then be used as a source of fuel. It is also responsible for clearing out any debris, bacteria or nasties in your blood, and ensures that blood leaving the liver is clean. An unhealthy liver (i.e., one that does not function properly), can lead to abnormal metabolism of fats, resulting in increased levels of blood LDL and triglycerides, a build up of fat in other organs, a fatty liver itself, and fat gain in general. Other issues may include sugar cravings, feeling sick, headaches and irritable bowel symptoms.

In order to optimise your fat loss and overall health, liver function needs to be a priority. Since most liver dysfunction can be a result of poor dietary habits (such as consuming too many fatty, processed and sugary foods), removing them is the obvious strategy to begin with. As is, removing excessive amounts of alcohol and other toxins (like prescription medications, chemicals and additives).

One of the best ways to support the liver is by staying well hydrated. This, in conjunction with quality eating and training, will ensure the liver is able to complete its detoxification processes.

Another important connection between hydration and fat loss is the mechanism of thirst. As mentioned previously, if someone is in a chronic state of dehydration, their thirst response becomes blunted; however, they may actually eat more because they think they are hungry, when in fact they are actually thirsty. By remaining hydrated you will decrease the overall amount of calories that you consume because the need to eat due to a faulty thirst mechanism will be removed.

Drinks such as coffee, alcohol, tea and fizzy drinks fall collectively under the name 'diuretics'. You may have noticed that your need to go to the bathroom increases with the more of these you consume (this is particularly true of alcohol). As such, it is important to keep yourself hydrated by drinking a glass of water for every one of these that you consume.

KEY POINTS

1. Hydration is crucial for fat loss and health.
2. Coffee, tea, alcohol and fizzy drinks are diuretics. They all cause dehydration so their intake should be limited.
3. Dehydration can sometimes be mistaken for hunger.
4. Try and drink at least six glasses of water per day.

KEVIN'S STORY

Kevin's biggest vice was fizzy drinks. He loved to drink them and would do so everyday – at least two litres! He would often skip breakfast, and he'd only eat lunch if his girlfriend bought it to him. At work he would have his trusty fizzy drink by his side, giving him the false energy bursts he needed to make it through the day. It's no surprise, therefore, that because dinner was his first actual sit-down meal of the day, he'd overeat every night (which, of course, led to constant fat gains).

One of the biggest issues with Kev's night meals (apart from the fact that they were poor quality and ill-timed) was his portion size. In his words, 'I would eat supersized portions. Everything was purchased and cooked in 1kg batches, so if I was making a chicken schnitzel, I'd make a kilogram's worth, even though there were only three people. And I'd eat all the leftovers so as not to waste it. Then, after dinner, the dessert would come out, and instead of limiting myself to just one ice cream, for example, I would eat the whole box.' And the same could be said when it came to lollies, crisps, McDonalds and all sorts of other non-real foods.

Since Kev was not eating during the day, his energy levels were exceptionally low, to the point that he often used to doze off at work. He was constantly struggling to keep his eyes open and his brain firing. His overall thought processes were also typically sluggish and foggy.

When a diet consists of low quality foods and is without fresh vegetables (Kev used to hate vegetables!), the digestive system is put under a lot of strain. There is not enough fibre to enable content to move through the digestive tract, and the body's absorption of essential nutrients becomes hindered.

Without this fibre, content and fecal matter can become 'stuck' and stagnate in the intestines, leading to irritable bowel-type symptoms such as constipation, diarrhoea, gas, bloating and irregular bowel movements – all of which are indicators of poor gut health.

Gut health is actually indicative of your overall health and since 70 per cent of the immune system is found in the gut, this explains why it's necessary to have a well functioning gut in order to feel good and be healthy.

Not surprisingly, Kevin was constantly sick; colds, sinus infections, and general lethargy were part of his everyday world, and his bowel movements were far less than optimal.

The huge amounts of sugar that he was consuming, in the form of fizzy drinks, were causing him to become dehydrated. Because this was the only source of hydration that he had, he suffered from huge energy highs and crashes, which were also was destroying his gut health. Not only did he look terrible, but he felt absolutely awful too!

The first thing I did with Kevin, to kickstart his fat loss journey, was simply reduce the amount of fizzy drinks he was consuming, while increasing the amount of water. He then gradually, over a period of weeks, worked on improving other aspects of his eating plan, such as eating regularly throughout the day, adding more fresh vegetables to each of these meals, reducing his portion sizes, and limiting the amount of processed non-real foods.

The results from these changed eating habits, speak for themselves. Not only has he lost the weight of two whole people, he is feeling vibrant and energetic. He has enough energy to get through the day, he has clarity and focus, is able to tackle gruelling training sessions and still remain active. To say that he feels better is a massive understatement.

Kevin explains it best when he says, 'If you eat shit, then you look like shit and feel like shit'.

TRAIN, SWEAT & PLAY

THE SMART MODEL OF TRAINING

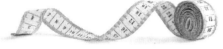

'What a disgrace it is for a (wo)man to grow old without ever seeing the beauty and strength of which his/her body is capable'

— SOCRATES

To really rev up you your fat burning potential, you need to combine great nutrition habits with smart training. I specifically use the term 'training' here instead of 'exercising' because I believe that there is a huge difference between the two, and a distinction that needs to be understood.

You've probably been told to 'exercise more' in order to lose weight and get fitter. This seems to be a stock standard recommendation from most in the health sector, and while the concept is based on good intentions it really is another one of those 'fitness myths' that I need to clarify.

Go into any gym on any given day, or go down to the local park, and you will see loads of examples of people exercising. It doesn't matter if they are running, lifting weights, boxing, walking or playing tennis, they are all great examples of 'exercise'. The thing is, not everyone who is exercising is 'training'.

Training is a methodical, well planned, long term approach to obtaining a goal (in our case fat loss), whereas exercise is generic physical activity. Think of any elite sporting athlete – do you think they exercise or do you think they train?

You're right, they train. And they train smart and hard. The reason being that for athletes, a methodical approach to training is required in order for them to perform at their best. Every time they step into the gym, or onto the field, or have a conditioning session, they know *exactly* what the goal is for that session, as well as the overall goal of their training plan. They also know *exactly* what intensity and effort they need to put in, in order to achieve their outcomes. More often than not, the type of training they do consists of weight training to help build strength and power, and high intensity training like intervals, sprints and circuits – all of which have a positive effect on their hormonal system (and body fat levels). This type of training enables them to have low body fat levels, and high amounts of muscle – exactly what a fat burning machine is made up of.

Now don't get me wrong. I'm not saying that there is anything bad about exercising; in fact, generic exercise has a large variety of health benefits and should still be conducted on a daily basis. What I am saying, however, is that exercise should not take the place of solid, intense training.

In the world of an elite athlete, every training session is recorded and outcomes are monitored, to ensure they are constantly progressing. Athletes are empowered and inspired by their 'why' or a 'special reason' that motivates them to keep challenging their boundaries. There is always purpose and mindfulness in their training.

The reason I'm using the example of an athlete, is because I want you to start thinking and acting like one. To make the long term changes that you deserve, you *must* change your mindset to that of a positive, focused and highly determined person – exactly like an athlete, and exactly the way the new, successful you thinks!

Bill Bowerman from Nike has a quote of his, sprawled across the Nike store in Manhattan, New York. It reads:

'If you have a body, then you are an athlete.'

Remember if you think it, you become it.

A well-planned, methodical approach to your training *will* see you achieve your goals, while minimising any potential injury, illness or motivational slump. And, most importantly, it will ensure that every training session you do is a quality one that will take you closer to your goal.

Misguided, unplanned 'training' becomes what I call 'junk training', and only serves to fatigue the body, predispose it to injury, and take you further away from your fat loss goal.

Similarly, 'exercise' is often performed based on how you're feeling on any given day. It typically lacks any real plan or programming, and the progress is not often monitored.

I like to refer to exercise as being 'undirected energy burning', or 'fun play' which, during the time of, will make your heart rate increase, help create a sweaty glow, and will make you feel good in the short term. But, and this is a big 'but', exercising haphazardly will *not* turn you into a fat burning weapon.

To achieve your fat loss goal, you must follow a training plan in addition to increasing the amount of incidental activity or exercise you do in a day.

INCREASE THE AMOUNT OF INCIDENTAL ACTIVITY IN YOUR DAY

There are loads of little ways that you can increase the amount of incidental activity or 'exercise' in your day. Start by reassessing how you get to work; if you are close enough perhaps you could start walking to work or home, a few mornings a week (or both!). Remember, there is not right or wrong here, the goal is to simply start moving more throughout every day. If you are too far away to walk and you take public transport, try getting off a couple of stops prior to your usual spot and walk the rest of the way from there.

At work, try getting up from your chair as often as you possibly can; instead of emailing someone in the office perhaps pay them a visit and ask them your question. Similarly, take the stairs instead of the elevator; volunteer to be the coffee runner and make a point of going for a walk during your breaks. All of these little blocks of activity will add up, and will have a positive effect on both your physical and mental health, as well as enhancing your fat loss.

Start identifying where, in your daily routine, opportunities for extra physical activity exist. Once you identify these, start acting on them! As I have already mentioned, small changes lead to enormous transformational changes.

THE POWER OF PLAY

If you have had the opportunity to spend time with children, you will have noticed their ability to play. Regardless of whether they are on their own or with others, they constantly use their imaginations to play.

Developmentally speaking, play is crucial for children as it fosters creativity, physical awareness, cognitive thinking and prepares them for adulthood. Of course, it's also fun, so with play comes much smiling, laughing and giggling. When I take my nephews to the park there is climbing, pushing, running and non-stop action; they only stop when they have run out of steam, and after a brief rest they'll resume it all again. There is nothing more joyous than watching kids engage their imaginations and become completely entrenched in their moments of play.

So why is it that as adults we lose our ability to play? The truth is, the benefits from play are just as important for adults as they are for children. Yet as we age, perhaps we feel as if we have to step into more serious roles, where play has no part?

Play brings joy to all ages, and it is important for our mental health, creativity and relationships. It can also be a great way of getting some extra incidental activity. For example, going down to the park to kick a ball around, playing frisbee or tag are all examples of play that are fun, and challenging. In New Zealand, there has been an initiative where local councils have developed a series of playgrounds that are both kid and adult-friendly. These specialised playgrounds include equipment that adults can climb, hang and swing off; no more watching children from the sideline – parents can get completely involved too! Other cities around the world, such as New York and Sydney are also installing adult playgrounds with the hopes of encouraging more activity and free play among grown ups.

Of course, you may find that dance classes or laughing groups are more up your ally; it really doesn't matter what activity you choose, just as long as you try to incorporate it into your week.

Playing will allow you to laugh and improve your mindset, which will have a positive effect on your lifestyle and fat loss goals.

KEY POINTS

1. There is a distinct difference between exercising and training.
2. Get into the habit of 'training'.
3. Use exercise to increase the amount of incidental activity in your day.
4. Always stick to your plan.
5. 'Junk training' is not productive!
6. Use the Fat Loss Method: train smart, train hard, train big, train often, rest well!

PRINCIPLE 5

TRAIN SMART, TRAIN HARD, TRAIN OFTEN

In the previous chapter I introduced the concept of Smart Training, and how it's a necessary part of your fat loss goals. Let me break this down further: the smart model of training includes information about:

- What days to train: training frequency
- What exactly to train: training type (e.g., weights, intervals)
- How hard to train: training methodology
- What sort of recovery is needed: within sessions and between workouts.

By following the Smart Model Of Training you will be able to get great results in a timely manner; whether your goal is to achieve fat loss in six weeks, twelve weeks, six months or even years, this model will always ensure you are progressing towards it. By sticking to the model, you will avoid injury and any potential plateaus that may decrease your motivation.

Smart Training is effective training, which means you don't have to spend hours and hours exercising, or playing around at the gym in order to achieve your goal. In fact, when people say that they spend more than an hour at the gym or working out, I know they are being completely ineffective with their time. Spending hours at a gym is not a badge of honour. This 'more is better' mentality that exists among exercisers, tends to be very counterproductive.

One of the benefits of following a well-planned training schedule, is that it is designed to get the best dose-response from the body (i.e., the body's best outcome from the dosage of particular exercise given).

Think of it this way: when you have a headache the instructions on the pack include recommended dosages, which includes a maximum dosage where anything more is not considered to be more effective, and – in fact – can even be potentially harmful. Well, the exact same thing can be said of over-training, or the wrong type of training. More is definitely not better! The correct type and dose of training will ensure the most effective results.

One of the most effective ways to obtain the correct training response is to train hard or, to use fitness industry lingo, to 'train at intensity'.

Regardless of whether you are seeking fat loss, muscle gain, or improvements in strength and fitness, in order to progress, your training needs to be performed at an intensity that creates positive stress on your body. Stressing the body is vital because this stimulus will, when given the right recovery, force the body to compensate, and then adapt. In the case of fat loss, training at intensity will cause certain hormonal and musculoskeletal responses that will encourage the body to draw on its stored fat for energy, and build lean muscle.

WHAT IS CONSIDERED 'INTENSE'?

There are many different variables that go into creating 'intensity' within a workout, ranging from things such as the amount of weight being lifted, or how fast you are walking.

We can use technology, such as a heart rate monitor to track the working heart rate and intensity during activities. Or we can us the Perceived Rating of Exertion (PRE) Scale, which is a subjective rating scale of 0 to 10 that you use to describe how you are feeling during any activity. '0' would be the intensity for sitting on the couch watching TV, while '10' would be you giving your absolute maximum effort.

During training you can manipulate the intensity by either decreasing or increasing the challenge of the activity, in order to hit the required intensity. Research has shown that once someone becomes familiar with the feelings of each of the different numbers on the scale, it can be a good estimator of their actual heart rate, and, therefore, intensity. With that in mind, the PRE Scale is, obviously, the cheap option to effectively monitor your intensity.

Both of these methods are fantastic at helping you find the appropriate 'intensity' for your training.

Training intensity is often referred to as being either 'low', 'moderate' or 'high', and working out your intensity is typically based around your maximum heart rate. The formula for calculating your theoretical maximum heart rate (MHR) is:

220 less your age. From this number you can then calculate your required heart rates based on your training zones.

INTENSITY TABLE

	% MHR	PRE #	TYPICAL DURATION	FEELS LIKE:
"Red Lining" Maximum efforts	>90%	9-10	2 mins or less	Completely out of breath, unable to talk, feel sick. Ouch!
Hard/High	>80-90%	7-8	2-10 mins	Difficult to maintain, uncomfortable. Breathing very laboured. Hard work!
Moderate	60-80%	5-6	5-6 mins	Sweating, slightly uncomfortable but can still talk. Getting Harder!
Low	<60%	4	indefinite	Light work. Moving and breathing easy. Not a problem!

If we were using your heart rate as the guide, then a high intensity would be considered activities that pushed your heart rate over 80 per cent or your theoretical maximum heart rate. At this sort of intensity you are working pretty hard, gasping for air, and certainly feeling it in your body. If you happen to be working at an even higher end of this spectrum, for example around 90 to 95 per cent, you would be what I call 'red lining'. Let me use your car as an example here. When you are 'red lining' it, you have got the revs up super high; the foot is flat on the accelerator and you are flying by at top speeds. Driving at the red line in a car, equates to fast performance, but it is also occurring at the expense of the fuel in the car. More fuel is used, and depleted quicker, so the ability to continue performing at that high level is somewhat limited, even though it is effective in the short term.

'Moderate intensity' refers to working between 60 to 80 per cent of your maximum heart rate, and is often the zone that makes you feel uncomfortable, although at the 60 per cent end it's still possible to have a conversation. There may be moments when you are gasping for air, or the body starts to feel challenged, but for the most part you could probably perform at this intensity for a sustained period of time. This intensity is the same as a 'cruising' speed in a car.

'Low intensity' is exactly that – anything that is below 60 per cent of your maximum heart rate and, for most people, this is the equivalent of walking and performing everyday activities. We could perform at this speed indefinitely – in a car this would be the same as crawling at a snail's pace.

The 'zone' or intensity in which you train will have a direct effect on your ability to lose fat.

For years we have been told that in order to lose fat one must train for long periods of time at a low intensity, as this is the 'optimal fat burning zone'. This, however, is just another fitness myth, because we now know that the most effective way to lose fat and increase fitness is to train at high intensity.

The closer you are to 'red lining', the shorter the workout will be, and the better the fat burning outcome. Training at higher intensities will promote the metabolic changes needed to allow your body to tap into its fat stores as a fuel source, as well as creating the positive hormonal profile needed for continued fat loss, blood sugar stabilisation, appetite regulation and muscle building. The best methods for creating this intensity is carefully planned weight sessions and interval training.

In the absence of intensity training, low intensity steady-state cardiovascular-based sessions such as running or bike riding for long periods will simply not cut it! In fact, it can work against you and actually promote fat gain.

The reason for this goes back to the dose-response mechanism I discussed earlier. Loads of cardio training does not affect the body the way that we need it to, in order to shed fat. That's because this style of training causes certain hormonal changes in the body that actually increase fat storage, promote systemic inflammation and contribute to the breakdown of muscle tissue. In this scenario it is easy to see why lots of cardio does not work for fat loss; however, many people still believe in the 'more is better' philosophy (but it's simply not true).

WHEN TO USE LOW INTENSITY TRAINING

There is a definite time and place to use low intensity training, and that is usually on recovery days or after dinner each night.

Aerobic-based training, or 'cardio' in the traditional sense is good for mental health as well as physical health. Aerobic-based training is considered heart protective (i.e., good for heart health).

Walking is one of the most underrated tools we have available; it is easy to perform and a good way to add more movement into the day. For the purpose of this Fat Loss Process it is recommended that a long evening walk (around 40 to 60 minutes) is added after dinner at least three times per week.

TRAIN OFTEN

Humans are designed to move in a variety of ways, and we are also designed to move often, however today we as a society in general, are pretty lazy!

The days of having to hunt, grow and gather our food or travel on foot to a neighbouring village are nothing but stories told in history books. Social conveniences such as transport, chairs, supermarkets, escalators, washing machines and the like all mean that we have drastically reduced the amount of activity in our day. Couple this with access to energy-rich food and drinks, as well as poor nutrition in general, and it equates to disaster – in the form of an overweight, sick and lazy nation.

Think about your own life for a moment. Calculate how much of your day is spent sitting down. When you wake up in the morning, and you've showered and gotten ready, where do you go to eat? How do you get to work? Once at work, how long do you sit down for? How do you get home from work, and then, when home, how much time to you spend 'relaxing' in front of the TV? Of course, after your exhausting day you go to bed and lie down. So out of a possible 24-hour day (of which we can assume eight is spent asleep), it can be 'guesstimated' that probably 12 to 14 hours is spent on your laurels.

This assessment proves two very good points:

- You certainly can make the time every day to train
- You need to increase the amount of activity in your day to even 'break even' with the amount of food that is being consumed.

Revised recommendations from the American Council of Sports Medicine suggest that people should be participating in a total of 150 minutes of moderate to vigorous activity per week, as well as two to three full bodyweight session. While that may seem a lot, keep in mind these recommendations are the baseline recommendations for maintaining general health, which means if you want to lose fat then the amount and quality of training needs to be more than this.

KEY POINTS

1. Stick to the Smart Model Of Training: Train hard, train often, rest well.
2. Your fat loss success depends on the intensity in which you train.
3. High intensity training such as interval training or weight training will create the best hormonal environment for fat loss, muscle gain and fitness.
4. Never rely *solely* on long low intensity cardio training for fat loss – it doesn't work and is a waste of your time.
5. Keep your workouts short in duration (45 minutes or less) and high in intensity.

TRAIN BIG

Any traditional training plan will divide a session into cardio training and weight training, with the cardio component typically involving 'huffy puffy' type activities such as running, walking, cross-training and rowing. Around the world it seems mutually agreed that people 'do cardio' to improve general fitness and weight loss, while weight training is reserved for those who are serious about 'putting on some muscle and getting big'.

For many, the mere thought of the word 'cardio' conjures up images of people slogging it out on a treadmill or bouncing up and down in a Zumba class; while the notion of 'weights' conjures up images of big beefy men grunting it out and dropping dumbbells on the ground.

Of course, neither are accurate. Weight training can be considered cardio, and cardio can be considered weight training – the labelling of these activities has long been misguided. We can actually blame the early aerobics 'lycra-loving, leg-warmer-wearing' pioneers of the early 1980s for this misconception!

The word 'cardio' is actually an abbreviated word for 'cardiovascular', meaning 'heart'. And any movement that raises the heart rate is considered 'cardio' in nature. Improving your cardiovascular fitness is vital for long term health and is also a key component for fat loss.

The stronger your heart is, the more efficient it will be at pumping blood around your body and supplying precious oxygen to the muscles and organs that need it. Just like any muscle, the heart needs to be trained too. Which brings me back to weight training – lifting weights does and will have both a cardio and fat burning effect, especially when performed in a specific way.

BIG BANG TRAINING

'Big Bang' or 'bang for your buck' training falls under the Smart Method Of Training, and it refers to workouts that use the big muscle groups of the body. You may also have heard the terms 'compound' or 'whole body moves', and they all mean the same thing: they use multiple joints and multiple muscles simultaneously. Movements such as squats, deadlifts, step ups, push ups, chin ups and pull exercises are examples of Big Bang moves.

Multi-muscle movements give you greater 'bang for your buck' in that there are multiple benefits to using them, more so then isolated movements that are small in nature, such as bicep curls, tricep dips, leg extension and so on. This is not to say that smaller, more isolated moves do not have their place; they can be useful, however if fat loss is the primary goal then it is best to opt for Big Bang movements.

Humans are designed to move; we are not designed to spend long periods of time sitting at a desk or on the couch. Our body has been beautifully designed to allow us freedom of movement in multiple directions, and we have the strength, speed, power and agility to run, jump, dodge, climb, pull, throw, swim or do whatever we want to. We are hardwired to do so, and our movement is the result of an evolved brain that allows our joints, muscles, and fascia to work in a coordinated, harmonious fashion. As such, our training and the types of exercises we select should reflect this.

Big movement patterns, when combined with weights, are essential for shedding fat and sculpting the body you want. When more muscles are being used, it means there are more calories being burned. The most important part, however, is adding load to these big exercises, as this will significantly contribute to positive metabolic changes.

One of the most effective ways to train these Big Bang movements is to put them into a circuit-style setting.

A Super Strength Circuit involves three to five big exercises (i.e., squats, step ups, lunges, push and pull). Each exercise is performed in a slow and controlled manner for a low number of repetitions (anywhere between 4-8 repetitions), before immediately moving on to the next exercise. You only take a break once you have completed all the exercises. This style of training is intense and extremely effective.

When starting out, using your own bodyweight will be sufficient load to have an effect, but as you grow stronger and fitter you will need to start adding some extra weight to the movements by using dumbbells, barbells or kettlebells.

The hormones involved in this style of training will help you lose fat and improve your strength simultaneously; specifically: testosterone, growth hormone, insulin and cortisol.

Although testosterone is most often associated with male adolescents, or big burly men, both women and men have this sex hormone. Women just have it at much lower quantities then men, which is why it is virtually impossible for a woman to get big and bulky like a guy from weight training.

Testosterone is critical for muscle development, body composition and overall feelings of wellbeing. As adults, low levels of testosterone can be associated with symptoms such as increase in fat or decrease in muscles mass, change in libido, mood swings, fatigue and lack of energy. Poor lifestyle factors play a huge contributing role to low testosterone levels, but improvements in these factors can result in improved testosterone levels.

One of the easiest ways to manipulate testosterone is by using the correct training techniques. High intensity training (such as intervals), correct weight training (such as the strength circuit) and quality sleep boosts the body's level of testosterone.

Growth hormone is a powerful hormone, responsible for the growth, repair and rejuvenation of all the cells in our body, as well as maintaining our metabolism (and therefore, how our body stores fat). Importantly, growth hormone is released in small spurts throughout the day, but the biggest spurt actually occurs in the middle of the night while you are asleep. Without quality sleep, both testosterone and growth hormone are greatly affected, which have a direct impact on both your wellbeing and the shape of your body.

When the correct type of training is performed, along with attention to the other elements, the hormones insulin and cortisol work in conjunction with testosterone and growth hormone to create a powerful metabolic cocktail. In plain English this means you create the ideal hormonal environment to gain lean muscle mass while also increasing your ability to burn fat; it's the exact outcome you're after!

FAT BURNING AFTER THE FACT

One of the most rewarding benefits of performing both strength training and HIIT is the physiological after-effect called 'EPOC', which stands for 'Excess Post-Exercise Oxygen Consumption'.

During training a number of complicated processes occur in your body, which result in the creation of an oxygen deficit. Once training has been completed the body needs to repair itself and replenish its energy stores. This process results in an increase in metabolism and fuel usage. In other words, you remain a fat burning weapon for a couple of hours after that workout!

Interestingly, the EPOC effect tends to be less high after aerobic workouts, which confirms that strength training and interval training are the most effective ways to burn fat.

SHORT AND SHARP

You may have noticed earlier on, that I used the phrase 'HIIT' or 'high intensity interval training' to describe a particular way of firing up your fat burning potential. HIIT is a very popular training methodology that promotes serious fat burning, improvement in fitness and the best part is, it's very time-efficient because it can be conducted in a very short period of time.

'Finding time' is often a big roadblock to exercise, but it doesn't actually need to be.

As I mentioned earlier, when a training session is conducted at a high intensity, they will be short in duration (less than 45 minutes). HIIT can be even shorter than that; in fact, some sessions only last ten minutes!

Normally interval training is conducted using cyclic type

movements such as sprinting, fast walks, stair running/ walking, cycling, rowing, swimming, and sled pushing or pulling. This is because they are typically easier to perform at higher intensities and they do not require a high level of skill to execute.

Interval training consists of distinct periods of work followed by a period of recovery, which is normally expressed as a ratio. For example 1:1, 1:2, 1:4, with the first number being the work interval and the second being the recovery interval. An example of this would be running up a flight of stairs for 20 seconds, followed by two minutes (120 seconds) of recovery (1:6 ratio); or walking as fast as possible between 4 lampposts with 8 lampposts for recovery (1:2).

Each 'work' interval needs to be performed at over 80 per cent of your maximum heart rate (or in other words, at an 8 on the PRE Scale), and the recovery needs to be an active recovery. Active recovery means being active while you 'rest' (e.g., walking, a light jog, or dynamic movement), as opposed to sitting still to recover.

As the name suggests, HIIT is intense, and does require a certain amount of focus and determination to get through each session. Performing at these high intensities can feel very uncomfortable, and probably well out of your comfort zone. Not surprisingly, physically exerting yourself at these levels can bring on symptoms such as rapid breathing, breathlessness, jelly legs, slight nausea and dizziness (of course, these will vary among individuals).

Ok, so I completely understand if you've just read this passage and are now wondering 'Who would ever voluntarily do something to themselves that would bring on pain?' Further on in this book I'll address mindset and provide strategies to help improve your psychology. But in the mean time, let's take a quick look at the concept of pain.

For a long time the 'no pain, no gain' mentality was a mantra for gym goers in the early 1980s. Jane Fonda, in all of her lycra-wearing wonder, would often preach to her audience the 'no pain, no gain' catchphrase, which insinuated that no gain would ever be achieved without an element of pain (above and beyond what was considered normal). This expression was quickly indoctrinated into the sporting and fitness worlds where competiveness and ego popularised it even more. Soon enough it seemed that experiencing pain was the only rightful way to earn results. The origin of the meaning actually dates back further than the 80s to the early 1700s when the then US president Benjamin Franklin was quoted as saying 'there are no gains without pains'. Essentially what he was getting at was that in order to achieve, or gain something there will be an element of pain attached to the process. It may not always be a case of physical pain (as Jane would have us believe), but perhaps emotional, financial or spiritual pain.

As with most things in life, if you desire something there will be an element of sacrifice and effort required to achieve it. In regards to achieving fat loss there are many pains that will most likely be experienced along the way. For example, the physical pain of having to exercise, the emotional pain of having to sacrifice going out to the pub with mates, or getting up an hour earlier to go to training. Transforming old behaviours into new habits (that will serve you better) can be a painful experience; however, learning how to view this pain as a positive experience and not a negative one will help you in the long run.

If you truly want to achieve fat loss and enjoy all the benefits that come with that milestone, then changing your perspective and learning how to experience uncomfortable and sometimes painful situations, will be a necessity. It is unrealistic to think that you can achieve your fat loss goals by staying inside your comfort zone.

It is important to realise though, that this uncomfortable, barrier-pushing pain is beneficial pain, and should not be confused with detrimental pain. An example of detrimental physical pain is if suffer from an injury, such as a pulled muscle.

One of the best ways to overcome your fear of pain is to get comfortable with being uncomfortable. Of course, this holds true for any area of your life – if you want to get a promotion at work, find yourself a partner, or learn something new, in doing so you will need to venture outside the familiar and expand your current comfort zone boundaries.

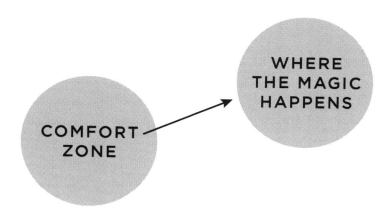

There is no way around it. To truly move into a place where you can transform your life you will need to take a leap of faith and get out of your comfort zone.

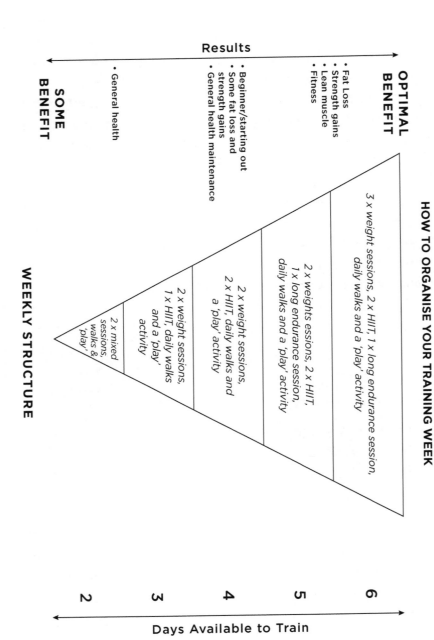

HOW TO ORGANISE YOUR TRAINING WEEK

OPTIMAL BENEFIT

- Fat Loss
- Strength gains
- Lean muscle
- Fitness

- Beginner/starting out
- Some fat loss and strength gains
- General health maintenance

- General health

SOME BENEFIT

Results

3 x weight sessions, 2 x HIIT, 1 x long endurance session, daily walks and a 'play' activity

2 x weights essions, 2 x HIIT, 1 x long endurance session, daily walks and a 'play' activity

2 x weight sessions, 2 x HIIT, daily walks and a 'play' activity

2 x weight sessions, 1 x HIIT, daily walks and a 'play' activity

2 x mixed sessions, walks & 'play'

WEEKLY STRUCTURE

6

5

4

3

2

Days Available to Train

KEY POINTS

1. HIIT stands for High Intensity Interval Training.
2. Intervals describe work to rest ratios.
3. Work intervals are designed to be performed at over 80 per cent maximum heart rate (MaxHR).
4. Active recovery is needed between each interval.
5. Some physical pain is completely okay, and is necessary for change.
6. Growth occurs outside your comfort zone.

KEVIN'S STORY

When we first started working together, one of the major barriers and considerations was Kevin's physical size. His movement was impaired, so doing simple little tasks was a struggle. Not only did his muscles and joints feel the impact of carrying 200+kg, his overall fitness was poor, and his tolerance to exercise was extremely low (as you would expect).

Just thinking about exercise was a scary thought, let alone the concept of 'training like an athlete', but from day one, we were determined to achieve his fat loss goals, and this meant having a well planned, clearly defined training schedule.

Kevin knew what was expected of him, and every single time he walked into that gym he tapped into his inner athlete, got into the zone, and got the work done. Yes, there certainly were difficult days, where all he wanted to do was turn around and go back to bed, but he knew that in order to make the monumental change that was required – essentially to save his life – he had to stick to the plan.

Having a purpose and a strong desire to achieve his goals

helped keep Kevin focused and determined. And, just as an athlete does, visualising his success was also an effective strategy to maintain motivation.

GOING HARD

If I had a dollar for every time someone commented on how hard Kev trained I would be a very rich woman!

It was not unusual to see Kev and I together, me with the proverbial whip-like voice, and him red-faced and heaving.

Kev has a reputation as someone who 'goes hard', each and every single time he trains, and it is because of this that he has been so successful with his fat loss, as well as why he continues to be the fat loss weapon he is today.

Putting in the effort and sticking to the intensity meant Kevin needed to learn how to go to that place inside his head, where he can surrender to the pain and allow his body and mind to keep pushing through.

Kevin had to develop this skill, it was not something that came easy to him.

Kevin would be the first to admit that he was one of the laziest people on the planet. He avoided moving at all costs, so it was no surprise to find out that when we calculated how much of his day was spent moving, it totalled less than 120 minutes!

Couple his completely sedentary lifestyle with his poor quality dietary habits, and it is clear how he became the size he was. Of course, there is a downward spiral that exists in this situation, in that the bigger he became, the less he was inclined to (or could) move, and the less he moved the bigger he grew.

It got to the point where to avoid having to walk to his bedroom Kevin would simply sleep on the lounge on his 'built-in pillow' (i.e., the fat pad on the back of his neck, which propped up his head!).

Transforming this man's mindset is what enabled Kev to succeed. One of the first major barriers that he had to overcome was learning to trust his body. Like most people, Kev had a large disconnect between his head and body and, as such, he did not fully appreciate what his body was capable of doing, or achieving. He regarded his body as a nuisance, instead of the remarkable machine that it was designed to be.

I often see clients who disrespect their body by feeding it junk, not sleeping, or taking care of it, and yet they are dismayed when their body does not perform or look they way they would like it to.

If you treat your body well, it will reward you. Kev had to learn that with time and nurturing, his body would respond by losing fat, moving better, and by becoming fitter and stronger.

Initially Kev's endurance was low and he would tire very quickly. But in order for him to achieve his fat loss goals, I needed him to train as intensely as his body was capable. This was crucial for both fat loss and for his fitness in general. As such, a big component of his training schedule included HIIT, which we monitored using the PRE Scale and a heart rate monitor. However often we used whether he was smiling, swearing or giving me the finger as an equally accurate gauge of his effort levels!

Our first few HIIT sessions were low in volume, and over time as his fitness improved I built him up to both higher volumes and intensity. Initially, our intervals were 20 seconds of work, to two minutes of active recovery, repeated three to five times.

Asking Kevin to work at 90 per cent of his MaxHR was exceptionally challenging for him, not only from a physical perspective but also mentally. Having never really taken himself to that place in his head where he had to push so hard, really proved to be a battle. But, to his credit, he persisted and it certainly paid off in the end.

MODIFYING EVERYTHING

Kevin's sheer size proved to be a challenge when I was selecting exercises for him to perform. He could not fit on a normal bike, nor could he stand and walk on a treadmill as it was too taxing on his ankles. Every movement we did had to be modified to accommodate his physique. It's important for me to share this, because I know that a common fear among over-fat people or those who are incapable of moving well, is that they truly feel they just can't do anything. The truth is, movement can still occur, it just requires some lateral thinking and modification to make it happen.

The first time I ever placed Kev on a rowing machine, he was so big that he could not get his feet in the straps, nor move his legs due to there being too much fat tissue in the way. I modified this by placing a bench across the rowing machine, and only getting him to row using his arms. Did it look a little strange in the gym? Yep, but it meant that he was able to move at an intensity that enabled the proper dose-response.

Kev also had an extremely difficult time getting up after being on the floor. One of his fears was actually falling down while alone and not being able to get up. His legs and torso were not strong enough to lift his frame off the floor. He was able to do it with support, but it was still an effort. So, in the beginning, a lot of our weight training was based on him trying to move from a lying position to a kneeling position without using any support. And while you may not realise, this motion was actually an exercise!

Similarly, sitting his butt on a table and then standing

upright again, lifting his arms up in the air, balancing on one leg, and slamming a ball into the ground were some of the exercises I had him doing. While they may not fall into the category of traditional exercise, they were for him, sufficient (and effective).

The take-home message in all of this is that everyone has to start somewhere. And that 'somewhere' should be individually tailored to suit your situation. Just start moving and persevering with it, and eventually it will start to feel easier, and that's when the results will really begin.

RECOVERY

PRINCIPLE 6:

SLEEP, RELAX AND REPAIR

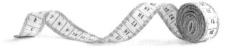

Rest and recovery are often the most overlooked and under-appreciated components of fat loss. Without adequate amounts of quality sleep, rest and recovery the body cannot adapt, and overall health and wellness will be compromised.

Proper nutrition, stretching, yoga, meditation and effective 'you' time are all perfect examples of rest and recovery. Very shortly I will explore these in detail, but first we need to discuss the kingpin of all recovery: sleep. Quality sleep, that is.

Deloitte conducted a study on behalf of the Sleep Health Foundation and concluded that sleep deprivation needs to be recognised as a severe health problem, as it is one that causes the country $5.1 billion in healthcare and indirect costs. Most adults need between seven and nine hours of quality, deep, uninterrupted sleep per night, yet many fail to achieve this, or if they do manage to get that amount of sleep, it is often poor in quality.

Healthy sleeping habits are necessary for a healthy body composition, optimum mental performance and health, and general wellbeing.

WHAT HAPPENS TO OUR BODY WHEN WE SLEEP?

When we go to sleep at night, it is like shutting down a computer. We physically rest our body, giving it the opportunity to recuperate. It goes through a process of both physical repair and rejuvenation, as well as psychological repair and regeneration. While we are in the land of nod, our body is undergoing remarkable changes – cells are being repaired, the musculoskeletal system is relaxed, and our brain activity slows down. Of particular importance to fat loss is the release and control of certain hormones that regulate appetite and fat storage. Human Growth Hormone (HGH), for example, is released in its largest amounts at night time (normally around midnight when the body is supposed to be in a deep sleep). HGH is one of the key hormones needed to maintain an optimal body composition. Effective training helps to improve the release of HGH, although the night time surges are the most effective. If sleep is hindered or broken, then the amount of HGH released is lessened, which then affects the total daily amount of HGH released.

A lack of sleep will also increase the hormone ghrelin, which will increase appetite, typically resulting in greater calorie ingestion throughout the day.

Dr Eve Van Cauter, an expert on the endocrine system and sleeping patterns, has concluded in numerous studies that a lack of sleep (e.g., six or less hours per night) is associated with the hormonal changes that predispose someone to both obesity and diabetes.

So, as you can see, trying to get more sleep each night will go along way in improving your overall health and waistline.

WHAT IS 'DYSFUNCTIONAL SLEEP'?

Although it is possible to function sufficiently day after day on dysfunctional sleep, we do so at a less than optimal level.

Sleep dysfunction is not just reserved for those suffering from insomnia (a particularly bad form of sleep dysfunction). More often than not, the symptoms of dysfunction are a lot less dramatic. Things such as not being able to fall asleep, waking up periodically throughout the night, waking up early, sleeping throughout the night but waking up tired, tiredness and drowsiness throughout waking hours, constant yawning and oversleeping are all signs that sleep is being interrupted.

It is also common for obese people to suffer from what is known as 'obesity related sleep apnoea'. This is a condition where you wake up in the night because you are no longer able to breathe due to the weight of your body obstructing your airway. In some instances this can become a life threatening condition.

Of course, in life, there are periods where circumstances will create disrupted sleep patterns. For example when flying internationally, having children or spending periods of late nights at work. Provided these are temporary events, catching up on sleep debt is all that is required. However, in a chronic or long term circumstance of broken, poor quality sleep, it can become a serious health threat.

One of the major reasons that people have sleep issues is due to poor sleep hygiene, which they may or may not be aware of. Many different factors can contribute to either improving sleep hygiene or making them worse. Good sleep hygiene refers to positive habits and practices that are conducive to producing high quality sleep on a regular basis.

Firstly, the type of food and drink that is consumed throughout the day will have a direct affect on your body's ability to shut down at night. Any type of stimulant (such as sugar, caffeine, cigarettes, or for some people alcohol) will release huge amounts of the hormones cortisol and adrenalin, which stimulate the nervous system. As the name suggests, stimulants will keep the nervous system 'fired' and 'buzzing', often at the expense of your night time sleep.

Unfortunately, many people rely on some form of stimulant to provide them with the energy they need to make it through a day; however, this potentially creates a vicious cycle that creates poor sleeping at night time, which reinforces the need for stimulants the next day, in order to make it through.

Technology has become a new type of stimulant. Although it has advanced us in so many ways, it can also be considered detrimental in other ways. Many of us are connected 24/7 to our phones, computers and tablets, with social media, emails, TV and games all vying for our attention.

Spending excessive amounts of time in front of these devices stimulate our brain waves, and at night time the flickering lights on the screens (particularly laptops screens) actually stimulate our tiny pineal gland.

The role of this tiny gland is to regulate sleep/wake cycles, and helps the body prepare for sleep by releasing the hormone Melatonin. It relies on environmental light levels to control this cycle. However, the bright lights used in your devices, as well as the LED-style lights used in alarm clocks, phones, and TVs, can trick the body into thinking that its time to get up, which is actually the exact opposite of what we want for the body at night time!

Additionally, a brain that is over-active is less likely to calm down for a good night's sleep. Thinking about the day's events, being stressed, worried, or hyped up from watching TV or playing games will all negatively affect the brain's ability to calm down.

A professor at my university once said 'the bedroom should only ever be used for sleeping and sex; nothing else'. He was right. If your sleeping environment is filled with distractions such as TVs and workstations, or other bits and pieces, then it is not an area conducive to sleeping.

The same can be said if the bedroom is filled with clutter and mess. More often than not, your physical home environment is a direct reflection of what is going on inside your head, and so a cluttered, messy bedroom, suggests a cluttered, distracted mind.

Noise, for obvious reasons, is also an environmental factor that can help or hinder the quality of your sleep. Limit the amount of noise that gets into your bedroom by using earplugs, or create white noise in the form of a fan, or a white noise machine.

Bedrooms that are on the cooler side are also more conducive to a good night sleep over those that are heated. Even though it may be tempting during the winter months to sleep with a heater on, for the sake of your sleep quality it is better to avoid doing so.

CREATE A PRE-SLEEP ROUTINE

Having a set routine that you follow prior to bed will train the body to get ready for sleep. Part of the reason for having one is so that you can start to unwind, physically and mentally, and allow the night time hormones to take affect. An ideal routine may look like this:

- 3 hours prior to bed, eat dinner and prepare food for following day (put kids to bed, tidy up).
- 2 hours prior to bed turn off all electronic equipment, computer, laptops, iPads, games and phones.
- 1 hour prior to bed have a bath or shower. Dim lights or light candles.
- 30 minutes prior to bed do some light reading, meditation, journal writing or gratitude routines.

NUTRITION FOR RECOVERY

Although we have discussed nutrition as it relates to fat loss, it's important to understand that it is also integral to recovery.

This is especially true the more physically active you become. When exercising or training, the body uses glucose, fat and protein stores as fuel sources. During bouts of high intensity training, the body relies even more on these good quality fuel sources. In order to replenish these stores of energy the body must get it from an external source – in other words, what you eat.

One of the most important times to eat for recovery is straight after training. There is approximately a 60-minute window to supply the body with nutrients, so that they can be absorbed and taken to the cells that need it the most.

During this window the cells are going through a phase of repair and replenishment, so it is in your best interest to supply the body with as many nutrients as possible during this phase.

Despite what you may have read or heard, not eating for prolonged periods after training will not speed up your fat loss. In fact, doing so will actually hinder your body's ability to repair and replenish, which will have a negative effect on performance the following day. Remember, a high performance sports car cannot perform if there is no fuel in the tank. The same can be said of your body.

Of course, the foods that you choose to refuel your body with are crucial. Quality nutrients are the primary goal and, in particular, glucose and protein. The glucose (sugar) is needed to help replenish your muscle's glycogen stores that have been used up during training, while the protein is necessary to help with the repair of tissues and cells.

To give you an idea of how important post-workout nutrition is for getting results, think about those supplement companies who spend millions of dollars designing and testing their formulas. Of course, many of these supplements fall into the non-real food category and so should be avoided, however, the point remains – nutrition after training is vital for optimal recovery and results.

You may notice, as you start increasing the amount of training you do, that your appetite increases. This is a good thing because it means your metabolism is increasing to meet your energy requirements. Keep fuelling your machine with high quality real foods, and you will notice that you have more energy and will be able to train harder during your workouts. The result of this will be an improved body composition and a giant step towards fat loss success.

EXERCISE AS RECOVERY

Yoga, Pilates, stretching, or general play is a great way to optimise your recovery. It is also the perfect time to add more physical activity into your week. One of the biggest mistakes made my people who are sore from training is that they cease all movement. But in actual fact, this can make you feel even sorer!

If someone is new to exercise or training they may experience what is called DOMS, which stands for 'delayed onset of muscle soreness'. DOMS may typically last from two to four days post-workout. If you have never experienced DOMS it can be alarming, because it can feel very unpleasant! Simple things such as sitting down on the toilet seat, brushing your hair or even walking downstairs can become difficult, but don't worry – it is a very normal part of the process. What is happening, is that there may be tiny micro-tears in the muscles you challenged during your training, and these tears cause a pain response. Funnily enough, the best way to help get through it is by moving!

Activities such as yoga, Pilates or other types of movements that involve stretching are the perfect solution. Not only will they physically relax the body, and improve mobility and flexibility, but these mind/body exercises have huge psychological benefits as well.

Of course, don't feel limited to these activities. If you feel like going for a leisurely walk, swim, a gentle cycle or an old fashioned play at the park with the kids, then go for it. All of these types of things count during your recovery – and they're all good for you, both physically and mentally.

Other ways to recover include massages, warm baths, ice

baths (yes, you read that right!), lying on a foam roller, and mobility sessions.

Remember, the quality of your training and how much physical effort you are able to put into each session, is directly proportionate to how much sleep, nutrition and recovery is obtained.

LOWERING YOUR STRESS LEVELS

We all have stress in our lives but, the truth is, we actually need stress in order for us to function.

Richard S Lazarus says stress is the 'condition felt or experienced when the person perceives that demands exceed the personal and social resources that the individual can mobilise'.

In other words, there will be little stress if someone has the ability or resources to cope with a stressor (the name given to potential stress triggers). Alternatively, if a person perceives that stressor to be too much for them to deal with, then a stress response will occur.

If we didn't have any form of stress in our lives we would never grow or become motivated to do anything. For example, the pressure of having to get up in the morning and go to work, or get ready in time to catch a bus, is one example of everyday stress. For the most part, we do not perceive these things as being too stressful, so they could be considered examples of healthy stress.

Another example can be seen when we consider our bones. The reason our bones remain hard and durable, is because of the daily stress created by the surrounding muscles and tissues pulling on them. Bones endure an ongoing natural process of breakdown then repair. If our muscles and the surrounding tissues did not pull on our bones and cause stress, then the rejuvenation process would not occur and we'd be left with very brittle bones. This disease, by the way, is called Osteoporosis.

People respond to stressors in different ways. Some may find skydiving to be an exhilarating experience, while others would be scared to death. Some find public speaking enjoyable, while others would rather chew off their own arm than speak in front of an audience.

How we perceive the stressor will determine how we react to it. This perception is based on our history, past experiences and our overall frame of reference.

To a certain extent there are always similar physiological reactions to stress, such as increase in heart rate, an increased breathing rate and a rush of cortisol and adrenalin. But there can also be individual reactions, such as nausea, headaches or breaking out into a rash.

Think about how you deal with stress in your life. Do you hold it in your body, and experience an increase in muscle tightness? Do you get headaches? Does your appetite increase or decrease? Or do you feel sick and jittery?

Short term stress, when dealt with appropriately, is nothing to be alarmed about. Chronic stress, however, can become a serious health issue, and is often a precursor for many of the health problems we see in our population today.

In order to fully understand why this is so, we need to take a look at our cave-dwelling ancestors. By the time Homo sapiens started migrating across the world, our brains had evolved to a higher brain function enabling us to conduct cognitive thinking, reasoning, tool development, ritual and culture.

In order for the species to survive, our brains also developed complex safety mechanisms. In particular, the 'fight or flight' mechanism. You may have even experienced this at some point. For example when walking home late at night, you hear footsteps behind you. In response, you may have felt the hairs on the back of your neck rise, your heart rate and breathing quickens, and your body tenses in preparation for whatever may happen next.

This is an acute physiological response to any perceived harmful or dangerous threat and the same thing occurred for our ancestors (except for them it was normally the threat of an ancient tiger or something equally as big and scary).

Physiologically speaking, a flood of hormones is released, the heart rate and blood pressure increases, vaso-dilation to the muscles occurs (this is where the blood vessels become wider so more blood can be delivered to the muscles), and blood glucose levels increase. All of these things are designed to get your body physically prepared to fight the threat, or provide you with enough energy to run away from it.

Once a threat has disappeared the body returns to its resting state and life continues as usual. This response worked beautifully for our ancestors, because apart from the threat of being eaten or attacked by other large animals or tribes, there were no other major threats to perceive.

Modern man, however, faces a very different situation. Our brain cannot actually recognise the difference between a *real* threat and a *perceived* threat, and since our stress response is hardwired in us, we will respond in the same physiological way as our ancestors did to their perceived threats.

We are bombarded with a multitude of stressors on a daily basis. Every day we face emotional, financial, chemical, physical, nutritional, traumatic and psycho-spiritual stress. Things such as worrying about events that are out of our control, money concerns, coffee consumption, alcohol intake, medication, injuries, being overweight, poor eating habits, lack of sleep, depression, chemicals and toxins, are all common stressors that many of us face every day.

Stress builds upon itself and if not dealt with in an effective manner can lead, over time, to an intolerance of triggers that would normally be considered non-stressful. That phrase, 'it was the straw that broke the camels back' describes this situation perfectly.

Cortisol, one of the major stress hormones, is responsible for muscle breakdown and fat gain, particularly fat gain around the mid-section. This particular type of fat gain is widely recognised as being more of a risk factor for heart disease than any other location of fat storage. It is important to note that chronic elevated levels of stress, and it's resulting systemic inflammation are disastrous for your health.

Now, here is something that makes my Fat Loss Process unique from many others:

If, you are someone who has a lot of stress in your life, the first thing you need to do to start improving your health is to reduce your stress levels. In order to drop fat, you must remove your body from that constant fight or flight mode. Furthermore, if you embark on an exercise regime that is not well planned, or one that does not encompass the vital elements of nutrition, sleep, recovery and mindset then you will actually increase your stress, and you WILL gain more fat as a result.

This lesser-known fact is the reason why traditional weight loss strategies fail. In order for fat loss to occur, you *must* take a holistic approach.

In the following chapters I will delve into certain mind/ body strategies that will help you become better equipped to deal with everyday stressors, but for now lets look at a couple of simple, quick solutions that will have a positive impact.

Chemical stressors:

Chemicals are found in virtually everything that we use, from shampoos to make up, to drink bottles. As such, it would be very easy to say 'just avoid' everything, but that is clearly not realistic. A few simple changes, however, can have a profound effect.

Just like food labels, the more names and numbers on the back of products the more chemicals they contain and, therefore, potential toxins. Start by choosing cleaning products and beauty products that contain organic or natural ingredients.

Certain plastics such as drink bottles, cans of food and plastic containers, contain the chemical BPA (Bisphenol A), which is used to make the plastic hard. It has been found that these chemicals can leech out of the plastics and into the body, and this process has been associated with hormonal disruption, cancer, heart problems and changes in brain function. Prolonged exposure to these chemicals does pose a worrying concern to your health (with infants and children having a higher risk). Many companies these days are producing plastics that are BPA-free, but even better, you can stop using plastics altogether and switch to metal or glass containers, jars and bottles.

Nutritional stressors:

By embracing a healthy eating plan that is based on large amounts of real whole foods you will, by default, be lowering your nutritional stress.

Earlier, we discussed how non-real foods are harder for the body to breakdown and process because it is not accustomed to the foreign chemicals. Trans-fats, corn syrups, high fructose corn syrups, hydrogenated oils and the like will disrupt your body's ability to function.

As opposed to focusing on foods that you 'can't have', focus on the foods that you should increase. By approaching your nutrition like this you will always be in a positive mindset, as opposed to a negative, restrictive frame of mind.

KEY POINTS

1. The brain does not know the difference between a real threat and a perceived threat, so will respond in the same way.
2. Chronic high levels of stress will cause systemic inflammation, fat gain, illness and poor mental health.
3. Stress is cummulative – the more stress in your life, the more it will affect your overall health and wellbeing.
4. There are many different types of stressors, such as financial, emotional, physical, nutritional, chemical and psycho-spiritual.

MINDSET

THINK YOURSELF SUCCESSFUL

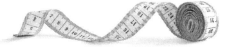

'People become really quite remarkable when they start thinking that they can do things. When they believe in themselves they have the first secret of success.'

— NORMAN VINCENT PEALE

Have you ever wondered why some people are more successful in life than others? Is it because they have more money, more resources and better connections than less successful people?

Certainly, money, resources and opportunities can help, but I would suggest that it has more to do with their mindset; or, more specifically, the beliefs and attitude they hold about themselves and the world.

PRINCIPLE 7

TO CHANGE YOUR BODY YOU MUST CHANGE YOUR MIND

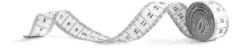

Your mindset refers to how you think about things; your own particular set of ideas and attitudes that determine how you approach your world. These ideas and opinions are built up over the years and are largely based on the experiences you've had. As time progresses these beliefs or attitudes tend to become 'fixed', which is why they can be difficult to change.

Take a moment to think about your childhood. Think about what your teachers, parents and others used to say about you. If you were constantly told that you were 'lazy, stupid, fat, dumb or useless' then you probably believed it and on some deeper level you might even still believe that about yourself.

If you repeatedly tell someone something (particularly during an influential development phase) then, most often, they will become it. And throughout life, certain events and experiences will reinforce that belief. For example, if you do not receive the promotion at work, you might think it's because you're 'too dumb'. Or if the partner of your dreams leaves, you might attribute that to being 'unlovable'. Or you may have developed stories as an adult, for example, you might believe that you can't lose fat because you 'have the fat gene', or because being over-fat 'runs in the family'.

But the truth is, these events most likely have nothing to do with the beliefs that you hold about yourself.

To tell yourself that 'this is who I am, I cannot be changed' is to rob yourself of all your potential. And trust me, there is plenty of potential in you waiting to be unleashed!

The secret to shedding the negative self-beliefs is to change your perspective, and this is absolutely possible, if you *choose* to do so.

For a long time, the medical world believed that once the brain was fully developed and matured it became 'fixed'. Fixed in the sense that every specific part of the brain had a specific role and function, and if that part of the brain was damaged in some way then repair was not an option. They believed that the capacity to learn was capped, and during our senior years trying to learn new skills or tasks was limited. That was, until recently.

The new concept of brain 'neuroplasticity' has opened up a world of potential, and the implications are enormous. Scientists have discovered that the brain does not actually become fixed, it has the ability to remodel itself, adapt and change in response to whatever stimulus it is provided. In other words, your brain can be rewired to learn new things and perform differently no matter what your age!

Of course, this will not happen overnight, but with conscious effort and practice you can become a new person. Your old stories, the ones that are full of fear, self-doubt, self-loathing, negativity, failure, or whatever you tell yourself, can be removed and replaced with positive ones. The 'I can't', 'I won't', 'what if', 'I should've', 'I would've' can all be replaced with 'I can', 'I will', and 'I am'.

LISTEN TO YOURSELF: WHAT YOU THINK ABOUT YOU BRING ABOUT

'Watch your thoughts, for they become words. Watch your words, for they become actions. Watch your actions, for they become habits. Watch your habits, for they become character. Watch your character, for it becomes your destiny.'

— FRANK OUTLAW

Our thoughts have a direct impact on our physical self, and what we think about we often manifest in the physical world.

It has been estimated that we have around 40,000 and 70,000 thoughts per day. We don't notice this many because we are often distracted, and the thoughts are filtered out; however, it is believed that about 90 per cent of those thoughts are repeated ones.

Now, lets think about those tens of thousands of thoughts flying through your head on a daily basis. If a stranger were listening in to your thoughts, what would they hear? Would they hear kind, loving, positive words about yourself and others, or negative, fearful, mean words?

Whatever you say to yourself reinforces what you believe about yourself. It also sets off a cascade of chemicals and hormones that will have a direct impact on your body. Not surprisingly, negative thoughts will set off a stress response (which we now know leads to fat gains), which can lead to depression, anxiety, appetite changes, allergies, food intolerances and much more.

On the other hand, positive, affirming thoughts will have the opposite effect. Happy hormones will be released giving you a sense of wellbeing, and contentment, overall immunity will improve, the ability to cope with different stressors will be increased, personal resilience improves and you will put your body into a state that is conducive for success.

The bottom line is, when you think more positively, you become more positive; and when you become more positive, you are more inclined to stay motivated and inspired to pursue your goals.

DREAM BIG – THE POWER OF VISUALISATION

I want you to imagine that you are holding a big, juicy lemon. You pick it up, roll into in your hands while inhaling its scent. You then place it on the chopping board and slice it in two. As you pick up one half you notice the juice running onto your hands, and the strong smell of citrus hits your nose. You bring the lemon closer to your mouth, and as you go to lick and suck the lemon you squeeze an extra amount of juice onto your tongue. You can taste its sourness, and smell the freshness as the flavours circulate inside your mouth.

So what just happened? Did you mouth start watering as if you were actually eating a lemon? Did you get that puckering sensation of your mouth as your body was preparing you for the sourness of the lemon?

This example demonstrates just how powerful visualisation can be. As you noticed, you had a very real, physical response to a thought inside your head. Your imagination created something physical in your body. Earlier, I mentioned that the brain does not know the difference between something real or perceived, and this is a prime example. By simply thinking about the lemon and involving all of your senses, your brain has been tricked into thinking that it really is about to eat a lemon.

For years, performers and athletes have practiced visualisation as a way of preparing their body for performance, and as a way of helping them to learn and rehearse skills. The process is fairly straightforward, and involves the person visualising themselves flawlessly performing the skill or act. When they visualise, they make it all encompassing – they imagine the smells, sounds and textures of the environment, as well as how their body is feeling and responding. It is like creating a 3D movie inside their head. The more detail there is in the visualisation, the more effective it is.

Numerous studies have demonstrated the power of visualisation quite convincingly. EMG studies (EMG stands for 'electromyography', which is a way of measuring electrical activity in a muscle) of different athletes have shown that when asked to imagine a particular performance or skill, the exact same muscles contract and in the same order as if they were physically performing it. What these studies show is that mental imagery, or visualisation, can produce the *same* physiological effect as if it were being physically performed.

What this means for you is that visualising a very clear picture of what you will look and feel like in the future, can actually help you achieve your fat loss goals. Remember, the brain does not know the difference between real or perceived, so even if you are not in the shape that you want to be right now, you can imagine what you want to be like, and your body will start making the changes required to get there.

Mastering your mindset takes practice but, as with any skill, the more you work on it, the better you will become.

HAVE CLEAR GOALS AND UNDERSTAND YOUR 'WHY'

Once you have created a powerful visualisation of what you want to look and feel like in the future, you need to create the action plan that is going to get you there. Visualisation is an amazing tool, but without the action steps to make it happen, it will always remain a dream.

To achieve your dream, you must set some goals, but not just any goal; you must set both outcome goals and behavioural goals.

Most people are quite familiar with setting outcome goals. These are the goals that sound like 'I want to lose X amount of fat, in X amount of time', or 'I want to save $3,000 for a holiday', or 'I want to eat better'. All of which are okay, but there are two important elements missing.

The first is the 'why' or the emotive reason behind the goal. Let's take 'losing fat' for example. Decreasing fat is a favourable outcome for many, but is it the fat loss per se that is going to make them happy or is it what losing fat *means* to them that will make them truly happy?

Common reasons why people want to lose fat is because they are lonely, lacking in confidence, feel unattractive, are afraid of not seeing the kids grow up, feel like a failure, or because they feel unworthy or undeserving. You may or may not resonate with these examples, but if you take a good look inside yourself and try to dig deep, there will be some specific emotional reason that is driving your quest to transform your current life.

Naturally, the meaning behind your goal will be different to someone else's, so understanding your own 'why' is important because it will help you stay motivated and inspired throughout your journey.

In order for your unique 'why' to become a powerful tool it needs to be turned into a positive statement. Instead of setting a fat loss goal based on negative thoughts such as feeling unattractive, or unworthy, reframe the 'why' so it becomes a positive statement, such 'I am deserving', 'I am enough', 'I am worthy', 'I am healthy and vibrant'.

This leads me to the second missing element.

In the example outcome goals I mentioned, there was no real *substance* to any of the statements. In order for your goals to be truly effective, your goal statement need to be powerful, with full sensory descriptions, and written in the present tense (even though the goal is not yet achieved). As we explored earlier, the brain loves visualisation, so once it has comprehensive details and clear imagery, it will set about to making it happen.

Additionally, having a statement goal such as 'I want to lose two dress sizes in six months' isn't the most exciting statement in the world. In order to stay motivated and inspired, you want to have a goal statement that is juicy, colourful and appeals to your mojo. For example:

'It is (insert date of goal), and I am (insert where you are) at my friend's wedding, surrounded by friends and family. I am wearing my dream dress (which is two sizes smaller than usual) it is red and hugs my body beautifully. I feel sexy, confident and full of energy. I am happy in myself and am proud of how I look and feel.'

Or, here is another one:

'It is (insert date of goal), and I am (insert where you are) at my office delivering a presentation to the staff. My suit is a size 44, which is the smallest I have been in over 15 years. I am confident and energetic and in control of this situation. I am happier in myself, and love the new level of intimacy in my relationship with my wife.'

The next step in this goal setting process is to come up with the actions or behaviours that need to be changed in order to achieve the goal. Too often, people forget this step, and only set the outcome goal, which does little to set the 'achievement' wheels in motion.

Setting these behavioural goals means coming up with a plan of action, which must be conducted on a daily basis in order to achieve the end goal. Small changes in behaviour lead to big results; or in our case – they lead to the accomplishment of the outcome goals that have been set.

Every decision that you make will either take you one step closer to your goal, or a step further away. Most of the time your long term vision and outcome goals are set for months or even years into the future, but behaviour goals are typically set for the present day. They can be broken into daily or weekly goals and are, essentially, the stepping stones to your outcome goals.

POSITIVE VERSUS NEGATIVE BEHAVIOUR GOALS

Reflect on your life at the moment, and think about all the little things you do on a daily basis that has lead you to this point. Do you drive everywhere and limit your physical activity? Do you drink alcohol every night? Do you buy takeaway food most nights of the week? Perhaps you hit snooze on the alarm clock five times before rising in the morning? A certain behaviour conducted multiple times becomes habit, and habits will either help or hinder your goal achievement.

Those who succeed in their fat loss journey are typically people who identified habits that were holding them back, realised how they could be changed and all the while they adopted new habits and behaviours.

Below are some examples of common habits that prevent fat loss:

- Drinking alcohol on a daily basis.
- Eating too many takeaway meals or purchasing food for every meal.
- Driving everywhere at the expense of incidental activity.
- Eating meals in front of the TV, in the car, or at the desk.

- Eating too much.
- Binging on processed foods such as, lollies, biscuits, chips, chocolate and desserts.
- Drinking too many fizzy drinks.
- Staying up late at night watching TV or playing with electronics.
- Eating when emotional (e.g., when tired, upset, angry, happy).
- Going for long periods without eating.

In normal situations most would formulate behavioral goals around '*not* doing XYZ'; for example, 'for one week I am not going to drink alcohol', 'I'm going to stop eating junk food' or 'I'm not going to miss a gym session this week'. While these seem like legit goals to work towards, they are set in the negative, and are about avoiding certain behaviours, rather than setting positive and approach-based goals.

You want to get out of the habit of talking about 'what you don't want', and cultivate the habit of setting the intent around 'what you do want'. Approach-based goals do exactly this; they focus on positive outcomes which, when performed consistently, lead to big changes.

Let's look at how to turn the above 'bad' habits into effective behavioural goals:

'BAD' HABIT / AVOIDANCE GOAL	APPROACH BASED BEHAVIOURAL GOAL
'I drink alcohol every night' / 'I'm going to stop drinking'	*'I will have one alcohol-free night per week'*
'I buy takeaway at least five times a week.' / 'I am going to stop buying takeaway'	*'I will cook dinner three times a week'*
'I drive everywhere' / 'I am going to stop driving so much'	*'I will take the bus to work every morning and walk home at least three times a week'*
'I eat all my dinners in front of the TV' / 'I am going to stop eating dinner on the couch'	*'I will eat dinner at the table during the week and allow myself to eat dinner on the couch in the weekends'*
'I eat when I am emotional' / 'I am going to stop eating when I get upset'	*'Instead of reaching for food to comfort me I will say "stop" out loud three times and go for a short walk'*
'I stay up really late watching TV/playing with electronics/ computer' / 'I am going to stop staying up so late'	*'During the week I will go to bed at 10pm'*

As you can see from this table, approach-based behavioural goals are based around taking positive action. Every time you achieve these behavioural goals you are creating new habits that are conducive to improving your health and achieving fat loss.

Additionally, these new goals are SMARTER – which is an acronym that stands for:

- Specific
- Measurable
- Achievable
- Realistic
- Time Bound
- Evaluate
- Revise.

The SMARTER criteria give your goals much more meaning. They also enable you to be clear with your focus, to measure your progress, to keep them attainable and within reach, as well as ensuring your goals are relevant, realistic and time-sensitive.

When you create your goals and map out your action plan it is important to understand that they are dynamic, and not set in concrete. Sometimes we set goals that are too easy for ourselves, and sometimes we set goals that are too hard or unrealistic. As such, we need to evaluate and revise them on a regular basis to ensure that we stay on the right path. Self evaluation or self critiquing is a crucial part of development and considering this whole Fat Loss Process is holistic, it relies on your ability to fine-tune your actions in order to optimise your potential.

Many think that achieving a goal requires a direct linear path from point A (start) to point B (goal) but this is not necessarily the case – in fact, the path to goal achievement can be quite varied.

By making constant evaluations, revisions and by recalibrating your internal settings, you will stay on track to accomplish your goal.

SUCCESS

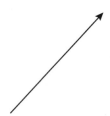

**what people think
it looks like**

SUCCESS

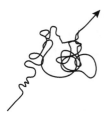

**what it really
looks like**

Drawing © Demetri Martin

KEY POINTS

1. What you think about, you bring about.
2. Your 'stories' are not the truth – they can be changed.
3. What is your 'why'? What is driving you?
4. Create powerful visions (this is your dream).
5. You must put an action plan in place, in order to achieve your vision.
6. Set positive, behavioural goals – make them juicy and sexy.

PRINCIPLE 8

CELEBRATE YOUR WINS

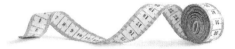

Too often I hear from clients, friends and even random strangers I meet in social situations, their complaints about 'not losing fat fast enough', or 'it's just not happening'. Yet upon further questioning and probing it becomes clear that they've actually come a long way in their fat loss process. They just can't see it or acknowledge it.

We can agree that keeping focused on your vision and dream is important, but so too is acknowledging the small wins along the way.

Every time you achieve a daily or weekly goal, it's a win. No matter how big or small it is, it still counts as a win in the right direction. For example, if you go from eating takeaway food every night to cooking three times a week and only buying twice, then that is considered a win! And every win is worth acknowledging and being proud of, because it is a positive change in habit. As you now understand, it is the sum of small changes that equals massive transformation.

Every single positive action that you take is allowing you to become the new person that you want to be.

Improvements in fitness, having more energy, better skin, improved immunity, better digestion, more mental clarity, and overall improvement in wellbeing are all amazing results, and definitely worth celebrating.

When you acknowledge these wins, the sense of pride and success will spur you on. A handy tool is to create a 'small wins' board. This is similar to a 'vision' board but, instead, it is an empty board designed for you to write up your wins throughout the journey. Every time you experience something positive, write it down and date it. It is far too easy to forget about what you achieve along the way, so this keeps it at the forefront of your attention and you can look at it every day for motivation and inspiration.

WHEN IT ALL GOES TO SH*T, PICK YOURSELF UP AND GO AGAIN

'I've missed more than 9,000 shots in my career. I've lost almost 300 games. 26 times, I've been trusted to take the game winning shot and missed. I've failed over and over and over again in my life. And that is why I succeed.'

— MICHAEL JORDAN

Without a doubt there will be times when things don't go to plan, or you experience failures along the way. This is a fact of life. But what will determine your long-term success is how you deal with these mishaps and setbacks.

It is very important to remove the emotion from any setback, and look at it from an objective point of view. When something doesn't go the way you hoped or planned, realise that 'failing' is not the same as you being a failure.

Failing means that something has gone wrong during the process; maybe you set a goal too high. Maybe there were things beyond your control that interfered with the outcome. Maybe it was the wrong goal in the first place, or maybe you chose the wrong action plan or it just wasn't executed properly. There are many possibilities to explain where something has gone wrong, but regardless of that you should feel comforted in the fact that everyone in life goes through similar setbacks.

If you choose to view a setback as an opportunity to learn something about yourself or your process, then you will generally find it easier to pick yourself up and power on. In contrast, if you choose to view your setback as a direct reflection on you as a person, and you interpret the situation as you being a failure, then the chances of you progressing are slim.

When a baby is learning to crawl or walk for the first time, how many times do they fail? At no point, does a parent, tell them to stop trying because they are not succeeding. We encourage them over and over again until they get it. The same can be said of adults.

If something does not go the way you intended, take a moment to reflect on why, and then realise what can be done differently in the future. Try seeing those moments for what they are: an opportunity to try something different. Just because you 'failed' it has no bearing on you as a person. You are not a failure; far from it. The fact that you are outside your comfort zone, attempting to improve yourself, and take on new challenges indicates that you are actually a winner. Setbacks are what help people improve and grow. The road to success is never clear cut or easy. Everyone fails at some point, you just have to dust yourself off, pick yourself up, and go again.

Sometimes though, the 'sh*t' really hits the fan, and it seems that *everything* you do goes haywire. During these times, I have found that the best way to get through these periods of craziness and uncertainty is to relax and just go with it. This may sound a little 'out there' but if you can allow yourself to surrender to the stress and discomfort, and simply let the situation run its course, you will eventually ride out the storm and with an open mind make decisions when the time is right.

Too often, when everything gets on top of you and the stress responses kick in, your focus and attention becomes too narrow. Your ability to problem solve diminishes. So, the more open and relaxed you can remain during times of high stress, the more likely you will be able to effectively problem-solve once calm has been restored.

KEY POINTS

1. Celebrate your wins, no matter how big or small they may be. It is important to acknowledge your success.
2. Create a 'wins' board.
3. Failing at something does not mean you are a failure.
4. When it all goes to custard, just relax.

PRINCIPLE 9:

CULTIVATE THE ART OF MINDFULNESS

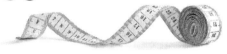

Ever driven your car somewhere but not remembered actually driving there? We have all done it at some point, and this highlights just how effective our automatic responses can be. Often during the day we will operate in autopilot mode, getting tasks done without really being aware of, or immersing ourselves in them.

Autopilot is a great mechanism for giving our brains a break; however it does not serve us well when it comes to fat loss or health. This is because in this context, another way to describe autopilot is 'mindlessness'.

Many poor health habits or decisions occur as a result of mindlessness. Have you ever sat down with a bag of crisps or biscuits to snack on while watching TV, and noticed that after a perioid of time the entire bag is empty? The initial intent was to only have a few, but because you were so distracted you over-indulged.

Overeating is one of the biggest barriers to fat loss and, for the most part, is something that can be fixed by practicing mindfulness. Come to think of it, *any* area of your life can be improved by practicing the art of mindfulness.

Mindfulness is the process of being completely present in the moment. It is an art that has been practiced for centuries, and it bears extreme relevance to today's society. When you are mindful you are noticing and bringing attention to the thoughts and feelings that are going on inside your body, without judgement. This is a particularly useful skill to develop, especially as it relates to your nutrition, training and sleeping habits. Doing so will allow you to gain control over your happiness and health.

MINDFUL TRAINING

In the training world we talk about creating a strong 'mind to muscle connection'. Every action we perform is the result of well orchestrated instructions from our brain. If we want to sit in a chair, the brain must send off a series of signals to all the joints, muscles and tissues involved in the process, prompting them to do their job. These signals from the brain to the body are lightening fast, and fall under the responsibility of our autonomic nervous system, meaning we do not consciously have to think about making it happen (incidentally, the same can be said of our heart rate, breathing and digestion). We cannot control these types of actions per se, but we can affect them by consciously making the effort to do so.

Any time you train, whether this be doing intervals or weight training, it is imperative that you have your head in the game. 'Switching off' is not acceptable and will hinder the results you wish to gain.

When training, you should be consciously aware of every movement. When lifting weights, focus on the target muscles being used and visualise them responding to the weight. Really concentrate on where the body is, how it is positioned and what is happening to the other limbs while the weight is being lifted. As a trainer, I am constantly reminding or cueing my clients on what they should be feeling, how they should be feeling, and why they should be feeling it. Bringing attention and focus to these details enables them to create a stronger mind to muscle connection, which allows them to progress at a much faster rate than if they didn't. They become stronger, more stable and more coordinated than their less aware counterparts.

During interval or high intensity sessions, when the heart and breathing rate start to accelerate you can use mindfulness to help calm the body. Quite often, in people who are new to this type of training, as the intensity starts to increase and changes in the blood alkaline/acid balance occur, the muscles start to feel heavy and fatigued and the pain response kicks in. It is a common response to 'lose breath', get flustered, or be 'unable to breathe'. This is the body's way of trying to force you to slow down, so that it can meet with the demands that you are placing on it. However, it can actually be controlled with mindful breathing. The conscious act of taking long, deep slow, controlled breaths in order to bring in more oxygen to the body, whilst removing excess carbon dioxide and settling the nervous system, will allow you to do greater amounts of work and, therefore, get more out of your training sessions.

This same breathing mindfulness can be applied to your recovery sessions, such as when you are stretching, doing yoga or going for a walk. It is amazing how effectively you can manipulate your body once you become fully aware.

MINDFUL EATING

Paying attention to how you eat is just as important as what you eat. As I pointed out in the scenario above it is very easy to slip into mindless eating which, inevitably, leads to over-indulging.

Mindful eating involves taking the time to slow down and fully embrace the whole eating ritual. It is often forgotten that we eat with all of our senses – our sight, smell, touch, sound and taste – and one of the benefits of being fully present during the act of eating is that we indulge all of these senses.

One of the best ways to practice mindful eating is to truly make it a ritual. Start by eating all meals at a dinner table; and yes if you have children, this includes them. Remove distractions such as electronics and TVs, and make it an experience. Set the table nicely, put on some relaxing background music and encourage everyone to take their time eating. If you are on your own, do the same thing – you are certainly worth the effort of setting the table for one.

In order to get into a state of mindfulness it is necessary to be relaxed. Now, I completely understand that this is not always the case, especially if you have been running around trying to get the kids organised, and dinner prepared after a big day at work. But it is certainly worth the try. One of the easiest ways to relax your body is to take a few deep breaths and give thanks. For some of you this may be done by saying Grace, for others it may be the simple act of asking everyone at the table what they are grateful for, or you may choose to give thanks in silence.

Before putting food in your mouth notice how it looks and smells. As you start to chew, actually taste what is in your mouth, noticing how it feels. Ensure that you chew all the food until it is liquefied before swallowing; this helps the digestion process and will aid in the relief of heartburn, bloating and gas. Putting down the knife and fork between every bite can also aid this process.

Eating in this manner does take a lot longer, but as a result you will be more aware of when you are full and satisfied (you can thank the hormone leptin for that), and you'll be less likely to over-eat.

CREATE 'TEAM YOU'

What do Steve Jobs, Oprah, and Big Kev all have in common? They are all superstars in their field, who have experienced great levels of success. Steve Jobs changed the world with his innovative combination of art and technology. Oprah changed the world through her humanitarian work and her focus on spirituality, while Big Kev... well he changed *his* entire world by losing fat and creating a new life for himself.

I have no doubt that their ability to achieve their goals relied on their mindset and hard work, but none of it could have been achieved without support. They each would have had a team of people providing support, guidance and mentoring.

People who make the best transformations are often the ones who have a great support network in place. It is not a journey that needs to happen on your own; in fact, by surrounding yourself with supportive and enthusiastic people you are more likely to be accountable to your actions.

Think about the key people in your life. Who would you like to be on your support team? It could include someone from your family, your friends, work colleagues or someone else who is going through the same fat loss journey. Or, you may choose to join an online community for support.

Sharing this process with others will allow you the psychological safety chute needed to keep you on track. In addition to having 'Team You', pick one special person who can become your 'accountability buddy'.

An 'accountability buddy' is someone who will help you stay focused on your goal. They will ensure you remain committed to your action plan and help keep you on track to succeed.

Typically, you will meet (or talk) with your accountability buddy on a regular basis, to discuss your goals, actions and achievements. They are there to offer you support and encouragement, but they are also there to call you out if you are not keeping up with your commitments.

KEY POINTS

1. Cultivate the art of mindfulness.
2. Be present at every experience.
3. Cultivate the art of mindful eating and training.
4. Create 'Team You'.

KEVIN'S STORY

Training Kev has certainly been a career highlight for me. I am so proud and feel so fortunate to have been part of this man's transformation. We have had many ups and downs and crazy moments, and among it all there is one particular day that stands out in my mind.

It was relatively early on in our training relationship, and on this particular day Kev was quieter than usual. I had decided that I was going to challenge him by getting him to push the sled, combined with some other compound movements. The session started out as usual, but it was missing Kev's typical banter.

He started pushing the sled with some force, but after a few meters he stopped. There he stood, in the middle of the gym with tears rolling down his face. This was not what I expected, and my immediate thought was that he had injured himself.

I asked him what was wrong, and he hit the sled (which is the same as hitting a metal pole!).

Though tears, and anger he replied, 'its too hard, it's just all too hard, the weight, everything is too hard!'

Upon further probing it was clear that Kev was having his first real 'breakthrough' moment. That moment where he realised that in order for him to be a success, he had to put all of his past fear, failures and negativity aside. He was at a point in his life where he had never been before, and the uncertainty of his future was scarier than the certainty of his past.

For Kev, in the past he was just 'fat and lazy' and that meant that no one put expectations on him, nor did he have to have any expectations of himself. However, he was at a crossroads, and by losing the fat and making improvements in his life, he was facing a very different, yet exciting future.

Here was a young man, who had never thought about what his future life could look like. Of course, he had hoped that he and Julie would take their relationship to the next level, but apart from that there were not too many possibilities on his horizon.

Kevin was in a place where he was exceptionally uncomfortable. Everything that was once familiar was now changing. He ate differently, thought differently and had a goal that he was chasing, but every step that took him one step closer to this goal, took him further away from his old self – the self that was familiar. He had two choices: to throw in the towel and go back to his old self, or to take a leap of faith that everything was going to get better, and to become comfortable with being uncomfortable.

While he was physically pushing his body, he was also pushing his mind, and in that moment of 'it's all too hard', his fears, anxiety and insecurities came flooding out. Fortunately for Kev, he was able to communicate all of this freely, and we were able to immediately identify his 'why'.

By the time we finished talking the session time had expired, but what we both learned in that 45 minutes shaped the way we attacked every day after that. Without that moment of clarity, he would not be in the winning physical and mental position that he is today.

That night I asked Kev to do some special homework. I asked him to start daydreaming about his future. He had to daydream with no restrictions, limitations or realism. He had to allow his mind to open up to any new possibility and these thoughts were what formed the foundation of his vision board – or as he calls it, his 'Get Sh*t Done' board – a place where all of his dreams and future goals are visually represented.

Nowadays, Kev's 'Get Sh*t done' board is a source of

inspiration and motivation. Whenever he feels low, hits a block or loses sight of his vision, he just has to take a look at the board.

WHAT NOW?

PRICIPLE 10:

TAKE ACTION!

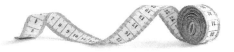

"I have been impressed with the urgency of doing. Knowing is not enough; we must apply. Being willing is not enough; we must do."

— LEONARDO DA VINCI

Phew, almost there.

You have successfully negotiated your way through a lot of information. The question that is probably on your mind, is now what?

The first thing to do is sit down and digest all this new knowledge. No doubt, there are bits and pieces of info that are floating through your head that need to be anchored and put into some actionable order. Putting the pieces of the puzzle together, if you like.

Successful fat loss is determined by your ability to continually take positive action, regardless of how small or insignificant you may think those steps are. Every choice you make will either take you one step towards or one step away from your vision. The more positive decisions that are made in the direction of your goal, the better your life will be and the sooner you will achieve it.

The old cliché of 'it's the journey not the destination that matters' is absolutely true in this case. Yes, getting the body you have always desired will be an amazing outcome, but what is more amazing is the holistic transformation that you, as a person, will experience. What I mean is that this Process will generate benefits beyond your physical appearance; your attitude, outlook on life, happiness, self confidence, belief and relationships will all change as a result. Life, as you've always known it, will be better.

One of my lifelong goals was to get to Base Camp of Mount Everest. For as long as I can remember I had always dreamed of being at the base of that mountain. But it always seemed so far away. Kathmandu is, after all, a very long way from New Zealand!

But finally, an opportunity arose for me to be part of a well led team.

We started our journey at Lukla airport (Nepal) and spent the next ten days ascending through valleys and mountains at the base of the Himalayas. The final leg involved a 4am start and a 7-hour push from Gorek Shep to get to Base Camp. We were at an altitude of 5545m and climbing. Every step felt like I was trying to move my entire body through thick mud. I had a screaming headache, was dehydrated, and struggled to focus.

After what seemed like an eternity, we arrived at our destination. The only sign marking Base Camp was a rock on the ground with the words Base Camp scrawled on it. One of my lifelong dreams was about to be recognised and the excitement I felt within was immense.

And then, I saw it. Another sign that simply read 'Welcome to Base Camp, 5,364m'. I looked around, taking in the sights.

Scattered tents, and big bins were everywhere. As I plonked myself on a massive rock, I remember my thought as clearly as if it were today. I thought 'it really is about the journey and not the destination because Base Camp is a dirty sh*thole!'. Sigh!

I got back from the trip a changed woman. All that I had encountered and endured had taught me something about my own resilience, attitudes and beliefs. The journey was definitely more important than the destination.

For you this fat loss journey may be your Mt Everest. Or, you may have another 'Everest' waiting for you elsewhere that hasn't revealed itself yet. Either way, your journey is just beginning.

The first step was reading this book. The second step is putting it all into action.

The following pages contain my 4-stage Fat Loss Process.

It has been specifically designed in a way that will optimise your fat burning potential and ensure you are prepared for long-term health.

Remember, losing fat forever will not occur using quick fixes or fad methods. Instead, it is the result of consistent effort, with small changes made across all the holistic elements of sleep, nutrition, training and mindset.

THE FOUR STAGES OF BECOMING A FAT LOSS WEAPON

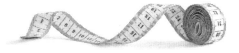

STAGE 1: LAYING THE FOUNDATIONS

Duration: 3 Weeks

Before you start implementation, it is important to take your physical measurements and photographs. While this may not seem appealing in your current state, it is an important part of the process because taking baseline measurements are a great way of objectively seeing how much you have progressed.

I recommend that you take girth measurements for your chest, upper arm, waist, hip and upper thigh, in conjunction with photos from three different angles: front on, side on and from behind. If at all, possible, a DEXA scan would also be ideal, as this will give you the most accurate measurement of your overall body fat, bone density and hydration levels.

In this phase I also want you to write a powerful vision statement about your long term goals.

For the next 21 days you will be focusing on just five simple things. Everyday try to:

- Go to bed before 10 pm (get at least 8 hours sleep).
- Eat 4 cups of vegetables.
- Drink 6 cups of water.
- Eat protein at every meal.
- Move for a minimum of 30 minutes.

That's it. Five simple things that will kickstart some big changes.

After 21 days, you will be feeling better, have more energy and be motivated to take it to the next level.

STAGE 2: GET SET

Duration: 4 Weeks

It is now time to up the ante!

The first phase was about slowly progressing you into new habits. The more time that you take to focus on habits the better off you will be in the long run.

This stage allows you the appropriate amount of time to adjust and accommodate your new behaviours. Before commencing this phase you will be required to set two to three positive behavioural goals.

During the next 28 days you should:

- Perform a kitchen detox – eliminate poor quality food items and organise your kitchen space so it is conducive to cooking on a regular basis (see Appendices).
- Keep a food diary for a week, and then practice measuring food (see Appendices).
- Work on scheduling your timetable. Invite people to be on your team, and find an accountability buddy (see Appendices).
- Slowly start progressing your training. Refer to the 'How to organise your training week' diagram on page 92. Start with the training frequency that suits you best (this should be towards the bottom of the triangle), and do not progress beyond 4 times/week).
- Focus on improving sleep hygiene by using the strategies provided in Principle 6.

STAGE 3: ATTACK

Duration: 5+ Weeks

During this phase you will be required to hit it hard. You will need to be determined and focused. It is in this phase that you will experience major fat loss. You can expect to see changes in your body shape and composition, and you will experience improvements in your energy levels, appetite, sleep and overall wellbeing.

During this stage:

- All meals need to meet the high quality, real food, portion controlled criteria.
- Monitor food cravings and language around your eating habits (see Appendices).
- Increase training to five to six times a week.
- Focus on improving mindset, by cultivating the practice of mindfulness and gratitude.

STAGE 4: REASSESS AND FINE TUNE

This phase is important for keeping you on track and moving in the right direction. Assess your current state by taking the same measurements and photos that you did in week one. Now that you have had time to apply your new fat loss strategies, you will be in a position to know what works best for you and what does not.

Have you been successful? Have you achieved results? If so, keep doing what you are doing because it's working!

If you have not achieved results then it is time to do some serious reflecting, around why not. Ask yourself the following questions:

- Have I fully committed myself to getting results?
- Have I given myself the best chance of success?
- Am I getting enough quality sleep?
- Is my mindset a positive one?
- Am I setting myself realistic behavioural goals on a weekly basis?

- Am I meeting the training requirement?
- Am I eating monitoring my food portions and eating high quality foods?

Answering these questions as honestly as possible will enable you to identify the areas that need to be improved. Taking responsibility and owning your actions will help you move forward and achieve success.

Once you have gone through a period of self-evaluation, go back to either Stage 2 or 3 and recommence.

You can repeat this Fat Loss Process as many times as you need until you achieve your results. For specific information on training plans and meal plans visit www.nardianorman.com

A FINAL WORD

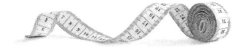

Firstly, let me say thank you, once again, for reading this book.

I hope that you have discovered a new understanding about how to become the fat loss weapon that you deserve to be, and are inspired to make positive and permanent change in your life.

I appreciate that leaving behind your old self is a scary and daunting concept. Change is unknown, so with it comes uncertainty. These fears are not just yours alone. They are the same ones that many of us experience and face on a daily basis. But, take a leap of faith and invest in yourself.

While no one can predict the future, I can assure you that by applying the principles in this book, you will be creating for yourself and your loved ones, a much brighter, happier and healthier future.

Finally, let me leave you with some advice that has helped me throughout the years:

- Continue to become an expert on you.
- Stay curious: apply information, test it, and change tact when required.
- Question everything.
- Keep chipping away at small behaviours – big change will occur as a result.
- Stay focused on your vision, but be prepared to change the roadmap if needed.
- Run your own race. There is no need to compare yourself to anyone else because everyone is different.
- Give yourself permission to fail. This is a normal part of the process and does not make you a failure. Just be sure to pick yourself up and go again.
- Surround yourself with 'Team You'. Supportive and loving people will be just as excited as you, to see you change.
- Ignore the negative, naysayers who tell you it can't be done. Their opinion does not matter.

Good luck!

Love Nardia

APPENDICES

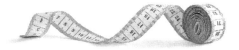

KITCHEN DETOX

- Start by cleaning out your kitchen and giving it a makeover. Grab a large garbage bag, and go through each of your drawers and cupboards and remove any items of food that fall into the 'avoid' category. The best way to stop eating poor quality foods is to not have them in your home.
- Arrange your kitchen so that has a clear space that is conducive to food preparation and cooking. Keep all your 'preparation' equipment in one area, such as cutting boards and utensils, and all your 'cooking' equipment in another area. If a kitchen has flow, it is easier and more enjoyable to cook in.
- To detox your refrigerator and freezer, empty all

the items out so you can see them. Bin foods that are old or do not fit the criteria, and take stock of what's returned to the freezer (this can be used at a later stage).

- Get organised: Place all loose food items such as herbs, spices, salts, nuts, grains into clearly labelled jars or containers (non-BPA of course). Arrange all tinned foods into a logical order in the pantry and allocate a designated area for each of your food groups.

FOOD DIARY

- Keep a food diary for a couple of weeks. Record what you are eating, the amount eaten, the time of eating, the location of your eating and whom you were with. Include all liquids such as fizzy drinks and coffee. This will help you accurately identify and assess your current eating habits.
- In the first few weeks of your fat loss journey measure and weigh your food. Take photos of the most popular foods that you use, so that you can build a visual library of your serving sizes (a good idea is to print them out and keep them in the kitchen for easy reference).

TIMETABLE SCHEDULING

- Write down your daily routine, and look for the places where you can schedule in training time and incidental activity. Print out this timetable and place it in an area where everyone can see it. Be sure to include three to six training times, daily incidental activity and at least one general play time over the course of your week.
- Consider where you will start your training regime. Will you buy equipment and train from home or will you join a gym? Investigate your options. Research local gyms, groups and personal trainers, as well as online programs or workouts. Find a method that will suit your schedule and budget.
- Invest in a good pair of workout shoes.

MONITORING FOOD CRAVINGS AND LANGUAGE

- Create a list of activities or strategies that you can apply if you have an emotional hunger craving. Keep this list in your wallet or somewhere handy that you can immediately refer to.
- Change your language. Pay attention to what language you use around food. If what you say is along the lines of 'I cannot have that', or 'I'll feel bad if I eat that', or 'I'm a bad person because I ate that', just stop. Remove the judgment from your

statements and rephrase things in a positive light.

- Pay attention to what your body is telling you. When you eat how does your body respond? What happens to your energy levels throughout the day? How do you feel when you are happy, sad or tired? Record these observations in your food diary or another journal.

REFERENCES

For a list of references please refer to my website www. nardianorman.com

EXAMPLES OF SERVINGS SIZES
(each item counts as 1x serving)

CARBOHYDRATES (vegetables)	CARBOHYDRATES (starchy and fruit)	PROTEIN	FAT	DAIRY	EXTRAS
½C cooked greens eg brocolli; beans	½C cooked coloured vegetables eg. carrots, corn	2 x large eggs	30gm nuts	200gm cultured yohurt	**Spices & Herbs** garlic
1x C leafy or raw salad vegetables, eg spinach, rocket, capsicum, mush-rooms	½ medium sweet potato	100-200gms chicken, turkey or fish	½ small avocado	200ml full fat milk	mint basil chilli parsley
	½C cooked oats, quinoa	100-150gm beef, lamb, kangaroo, pork	1tbsp ghee/butter/ coconut oil	2 x slices hard cheese	turmeric pepper/salt allspice
1 x C raw asian greens eg bok choy	1 x C berries (frozen or fresh)		1tbsp nut butter		cinnamon paprika
	1 x medium apple, banana, pear, orange		1 tbsp olive/ almond/apricot oil		**Miscellaneous** bone broth
			1 tbsp tahini		stock (homemade) almond milk
			200ml coconut milk		herbal teas

NEXT STEPS

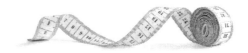

To continue your momentum I have included extra information and bonus material at my website **www.nardianorman.com**. If you haven't already go and check it out.

You will also find:

- videos
- exercise plans
- webinars
- 7 Week challenge
- access to seminars
- access to exclusive membership
- a community of like minded people all on a journey
- support and on going motivation

Also please feel free to visit www.fatattack.com.au

ABOUT NARDIA

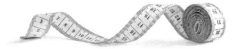

Nardia is an educator, speaker, author, personal trainer and health coach. Her life has been dedicated to helping people realize their optimal potential through good nutrition, smart training and increased wellbeing. She is a bona fide training and nutrition geek.

For over 15 years Nardia has been helping people from all walks of life to learn the truth about creating a body and life they love.

Tired of seeing all sorts of misguided information regarding Fat Loss, Health and Wellbeing, in conjunction with a passion for education led her to writing this book.

She is on a mission to change the outdated weight loss industry. To lead a new Fat Loss revolution in which the outcome is about effective, safe and most importantly long term changes in body shape that support optimal health and performance for life.

Nardia believes that everyone is entitled to good quality information that is simple and easy to implement. You will find her advice to be uncomplicated and immediately actionable.

When not writing, training or researching you will find her enjoying a glass of red wine, eating cheese and spending time with her equally geeky partner, Mike. She is also privileged to be a Champion for the Centre of Healthy Brain Ageing, a cause dedicated to spreading awareness of positive ageing and brain health.

BRAIN HEALTH

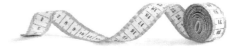

In 2012 I lost my beautiful grandmother to Dementia. Whilst I had heard of this condition it was the first time I had experienced it first hand. To watch a loved one lose their cognitive function, and then all function, is heartbreaking. Seeing my once strong, exceptionally opinionated, articulate Nana reduced to the personality and function of a young girl, was difficult. The worst part was during the early phase where she was aware that she was moving between the two worlds of clarity and lucidity.

If you have experienced this for yourself, or know of people who have, you will appreciate just how sad it can be. As such I was determined to find a way in which I was able to use my skills and knowledge to help; thankfully I found the Centre for Healthy Brain Ageing (CHeBA).

Throughout this book the focus has been on sustainable

fat loss and optimal health, yet every part of my process is also designed to have a positive effect on your brain health.

I am extremely proud to be a Fitness Ambassador for the Centre of Healthy Brain Ageing (CHeBA), UNSW Medicine. It gives me great pleasure to share the following information from CHeBA's Co-Directors, Professor Perminder Sachdev and Professor Henry Brodaty, and their Marketing and Communications Officer, Heidi Mitchell:

CHeBA

Are the scales finally tipping?

It is a sobering fact that there is a worldwide obesity epidemic.

According to the World Health Organisation (WHO), obesity levels have almost doubled since 1980. There are more than 1.4 billion adults worldwide who are overweight and approximately 35% of those are obese.

In 2011, more than 40 million children under the age of five were overweight.

Despite obesity being largely preventable, levels continue to escalate exponentially worldwide. The human body was not designed for such sedentary living and food abundance that we find in the 21st century. Interestingly, at the same time, the demand for health and fitness seems to be increasing, with more health clubs, fitness professionals and access to healthy eating forums and blogs than ever before.

Clearly something isn't working.

Possibly one of the issues with current trends in health and fitness is the attention on weight loss coupled with flawed attention on body aesthetics instead of a healthy body that functions properly.

Fitness Expert and Educator Nardia Norman has taken a grass roots approach to health in this book aptly entitled Fat Attack: the secrets behind the world's biggest loser. *Her book has a message for all of us, and it will hopefully act as a vehicle for clarifying misconceptions about weight loss and promote the indisputable link between cardiovascular health and lean muscle mass.*

Like all good books, it comes from personal experience. She knows the flaws in society as well as in the human mind, and knows what can be achieved through sheer discipline and resolve. The lessons she has learnt are applicable to all of us, and are particularly relevant as we face the coming epidemic of dementia.

Like obesity, dementia has rapidly become a worldwide problem, with an estimate that there will be 135 million people with dementia by 2050.

Importantly, the link between cardiovascular health and brain health is irrefutable and a major campaign has been undertaken by the Centre for Healthy Brain Ageing (CHeBA) to increase awareness of the modifiable risk factors of brain disorders to the general population.

Quite appropriately, Nardia is a CHeBA Champion. The CHeBA Champions are the Fitness Ambassadors for the Centre, and like Nardia are enthusiastic about increasing the understanding amongst their peers about the impact of lifestyle upon our brain health in late life. At the same time, they drive much needed funds to advance the research being done at the Centre for Healthy Brain Ageing (CHeBA) to prevent cognitive decline, improve cognitive functioning as we age and devise better care for people with dementia.

With the prevalence of age-related cognitive disorders such as Alzheimer's and other dementias on the increase, it is crucial to be aware that the risk factors for these brain diseases don't just point to genetics. Increased cardiovascular health, regulated blood glucose levels and a healthy blood pressure are all important components in brain health. More and more evidence is suggesting that up to 70% of age-related brain disorders such as dementia can be attributed to lifestyle choices in earlier life, which means there is a great deal we can do to improve our behavioural and lifestyle habits to strive for a better future for ourselves.

CHeBA is headed by two international leaders in ageing brain research (Professors Perminder Sachdev and Henry Brodaty), who, together with their team are working on developing markers of early decline in memory and other cognitive functioning so that brain diseases can be detected before the manifestation of dementia. The future of Australia will be impacted greatly by the outcomes of CHeBA. With an ageing population and at least half of the people in nursing homes with dementia, we need the high level research being conducted at CHeBA to facilitate long-term change.

Heidi Mitchell

This Centre relies heavily on funds raised from the Ambassadors to continue research. If you would like to help this worthy organisation you may contribute to my fundraising page, where 100% of funds go directly into the organization. Please go to:

https://cheba2.everydayhero.com/au/nardia

Also, on a personal level, of each book sale I will be donating 10% of the profits towards CHEBA.

Nardia

ACKNOWLEDGMENTS

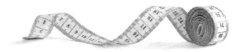

This book has been many years in the making. I have had the good fortune of being surrounded by many amazing people, who have, at different stages of my career either helped me, mentored me or been a source of inspiration. To thank everyone personally would require another whole book so just know that if you have ever come in contact with me then you have influenced me in some small way.

First and foremost, I have to thank my family for always putting up with me, and all my quirks. For providing me with unconditional love and encouragement, and for teaching me that I could do and be whatever I wanted to be. In particular to my Grandfather who taught me that there is no such word as 'can't'. I love you all.

Secondly, to my amazing, and equally geeky partner, Mike Campbell, for being the logical, calm and reasonable half of us. Since meeting you my life has flourished and I am the person I am today because of you. You are a constant source of strength and encouragement and without you this book would not have got out of my head and onto paper. Thank you for being on my team, for being my biggest supporter and for always making sure I have a good meal at night. Here is to our 'wins' board and future dreams. You are my meat muse, my best friend, my cook, my motivation and I love you.

To all my wonderful friends and colleagues that keep me on my toes, and keep me honest, I am blessed to have all of you in my life – my life is truly rich because of you all. Thanks for the laughs, advice and shenanigans that we have had and are likely to have in the future! In particular I would like to thank the kiwi kids who have been with me since the beginning of my career – we have all come a long way since our Les Mills Dunedin days! Dave, Steve, Hobbs, Muz and Ange: MYLLYM.

I have learnt so much from many of my friends, but one stand out is Susanne King who has been a source of inspiration, information and light over the past two years.

In addition I need to give credit to the lovely Leesa for being both my advisory board and proofreader in one. Your suggestions and help were invaluable. Also I would like to thank Greg Hurst, David Hatch and Lisa Chivers from the Australian Institute of Fitness for believing in me and giving me the opportunity to hone my presenting skills, even though I had a thick kiwi accent.

I want to express my gratitude to all my clients and students past and present, who have provided me with insight; good times and taught me as much as I have taught them. A special mention goes to Don McKenzie, my first ever PT client and my personal guinea pig.

Sometimes synchronistic events occur that change the course of your life plan, and one such time was a dinner with friends that provided the catalyst for this. As such I would like to thank Sam Elam, and Kylie Bartlett for giving me the encouragement and the drive to make this happen. We shall celebrate over bubbles soon.

Big thanks must go to my publisher Julie Renouf who has made this entire process seamless and timely. Thank you for taking me under your wing and explaining everything! Also, Analee Gale for editing this book in a remarkable time frame.

And last but not least, to the man whom this book is based. The man who has surpassed all my expectations and is now a shining example of what can be achieved with hard work, discipline and good humour. Kevin you are amazing, and a positive role model to all those who are struggling to make change. The world needs to hear your story.

Published in 2014 in Australia by Nardia Norman
http://nardianorman.com

Copyright © Nardia Norman 2014
Text copyright © Nardia Norman 2014
Book Production: OpenBook Creative
Cover Design & Typesetting: OpenBook Creative
Editor: Analee Matthews
Author Photograph: Simon Le Photography
Cover photo: Nata-Lia @ Shutterstock.com

Australia Cataloguing-in-Publication entry:
    Author: Norman, Nardia
    Title: Fat Attack : the secrets behind the world's biggest loser
    9781925144024 (paperback)
    9781925144031 (ebook : epub)
    9781925144048 (ebook : kindle)
    Subjects: Weight loss
        Reducing exercises
        Reducing diets

    Dewey Number: 613.25

Disclaimer: This book is a source of general information only. This general information
cannot, and does not, address your individual situation and so is not a substitute
for the advice of a suitably qualified professional who knows your personal circumstances. Because the information contained in this book is of a general nature only,
any reader who relies upon it does so at their own risk, and the author, publisher and
contributors assume no responsibility under any circumstances.

A medical practitioner should be consulted before beginning any new eating, exercise
or health program